APR - 2 1996	DATE DUE	NOV 2 7 2002
OCT 20 1996	FEB 1 2 1998 JUL 29 1999	OCT - 8 2003
NOV - 8 1996 MAR - 2 1998	SEP 24 1999	OCT 2 2 2003
APR - 4 1997 16	OCT 6 1999	NOV 2 1 2003
APR 25 1997 OCT 2 4 1998	OCT 29 1999	
JUL 1 0 1997		
AUG 0 8 1997 DEC 1 1 1998		
OCT 1 4 1997 JAN 2 1 1999	MAR 2 5 2001 DEC 0 3 2001	
OCT 1 7 1997 APR 1 2 1999	FEB 2 1 2002	
JAN 2 9 1998 MAY - 3 1999	SEP 1 9 2002	
JUN 2 3 1999		

*Women,
drinking,
and pregnancy*

Women,
drinking,
and pregnancy

Moira Plant

Tavistock Publications
London and New York

First published in 1985 by
Tavistock Publications Ltd
11 New Fetter Lane, London EC4P 4EE

Published in the USA by
Tavistock Publications
in association with Methuen, Inc.
733 Third Avenue, New York, NY 10017

Printed in Great Britain at the University Press, Cambridge

British Library Cataloguing in Publication Data

Plant, Moira L.
　Women, drinking and pregnancy.
　1. Fetal alcohol syndrome　　2. Pregnant women——
　Alcohol use　　3. Alcohol——Physiological effects
　I. Title
　618.3'2　　RG629.F45

　ISBN 0-422-78610-1

Library of Congress Cataloging in Publication Data

Plant, Moira L.
　Women, drinking, and pregnancy.

　Bibliography: p.
　Includes indexes.
　1. Fetal alcohol syndrome.　　2. Fetus——Effect of drugs on.
　3. Alcoholism in pregnancy.　　4. Pregnant women——Alcohol
　use.　　I. Title.
　RG629.F45P58　　1985　　618.3　　84-26773
　ISBN 0-422-78610-1

I dedicate this book to my husband, Martin, and our daughter, Emma.

Contents

Acknowledgements

My thanks go to Mrs Ray Stuart, my research assistant, without whose help the collection of these data would have been an even greater burden. I want to thank Dr Norman Kreitman of the Medical Research Council Unit for Epidemiological Studies in Psychiatry, from whom I have learned a great deal. Acknowledgement must also go to the many nursing, medical and clerical staff in the Simpson Memorial Maternity Pavilion, in particular Dr Philip Myerscough, and Sisters Isobel McDougall, Annette Paton and Grace Martin. My interviewers, Mrs Sheena Blair, Mrs Valerie Dunn, Mrs Dorothy Wilkie, Mrs Joyce Nicol, Mrs Lynn Steven and Mrs Heather Keith deserve my thanks for their enthusiasm for this study. The many health visitors who took extra time to fill in the development checks have my admiration of their commitment to their jobs; in particular I wish to thank Mrs M. Sinclair whose cheerfulness kept me going, Miss M. Nimmo, Miss C. Reid, Mrs J. Goodwin, Miss M. Hillier, Miss I. Marquis, Miss R. Watson, Miss P. Robertson, Miss D. Reith, Mrs S. McDade, Miss I. Tait, Miss P. Saunders, Miss I. Muir, Miss H. Brown and Miss B. Wylie.

Initial help was provided by the late Dr David Davies, Medical Director of the Alcohol Education Centre, Professor David Robinson, Institute of Health Studies, University of Hull, Professor Griffith Edwards of the Addiction Research Unit, London, and Professor Jan Kuzma, Department of Epidemiology, School of Health, Loma Linda University, California.

I am indebted to several members of the Alcohol Epidemiology Section of the International Council on Alcohol and Addictions for encouragement and support. Particular thanks go to Dr Ralph

Hingson of the Department of Socio-Medical Sciences and Community Medicine and Department of Paediatrics, Boston University, Massachusetts. In addition thanks for statistical advice go to the following, Mr John Duffy of the Medical Research Council Unit for Epidemiological Studies in Psychiatry, Edinburgh, Dr Ole-Jurgen Skog of the National Institute of Alcohol Research, Oslo, Dr Klaus Makela of the Finnish Foundation of Alcohol Studies, Helsinki, Mr Ralph McGuire and Mr Dave Peck of the Department of Psychiatry, University of Edinburgh.

The artwork for Figure 3 was kindly provided by Mr David Mason.

Thanks are due to Mrs Patricia Rose and Mrs Elma McDonald for speedy and efficient typing of the initial interview schedules and the text of this book. The librarians, Mrs Margaret Nicholson, Mrs Letty Chabot and Mrs Margaret Dawe were always helpful no matter how many obscure references were asked for. Many other people have helped with this study, both with their heads and their hearts, to them also I give my thanks. My husband, Martin, gave me support intellectually and emotionally; to him I give my love.

Lastly I would like to thank the women and their babies who, however unknowingly, made this study possible.

This study was mainly funded by the Wellcome Trust. Additional support was provided by the Alcohol Education and Research Committee and the Scotch Whisky Association. This book is based upon a Ph.D. thesis produced under the auspices of the Council for National Academic Awards (CNAA).

Introduction

The main concern of this book is the relationship between alcohol consumption in pregnancy and fetal harm. Patterns and levels of alcohol consumption are influenced by many factors, such as age, sex, occupation, nationality, and pressure from peer groups. Particular situations, such as social gatherings, also affect people's consumption of alcohol. Other factors include religion and changing roles, for instance, that of women. Pregnancy outcome is also affected by many factors, such as occupational status, age, parity, general health and nutritional status of mother, awareness of need for good antenatal care and avoidance of infections such as rubella.

The book's central aim is to identify the role of alcohol in relation to a constellation of possible confounding factors, such as legal and illicit drug use.

Current concern about the possible ill effects of drinking during pregnancy coincides with an upsurge of alcohol use and misuse among women. The levels of alcohol-related problems in a community are closely linked to the per capita level of consumption. An increase in consumption is invariably mirrored by an increase in alcohol-related problems (Peck 1982: 73). It is therefore relevant to address first the recent changes in women's alcohol consumption. It is clear that alcohol-related problems among women in both the United Kingdom and elsewhere, have been growing. One extreme indication of this has been a steady rise in the proportion of women among those admitted to psychiatric hospitals for alcohol dependence and alcoholic psychosis in the United Kingdom. In Scotland in 1970, 19 per cent of all first admissions with these diagnoses were women. By 1982 the corresponding proportion of women had risen

1

to 24 per cent. Cirrhosis of the liver, which is closely related to excessive drinking, has also shown an increase. The rate of deaths from liver cirrhosis in the United Kingdom has risen by 25 per cent in the last decade. The greatest increase in this rate has been among women (Thorley 1982: 49).

The most obvious reason for this upsurge of alcohol-related problems has been the general rise in alcohol consumption. Shaw, in a recent review, stated:

'In Britain women's drinking problems have undergone a more dramatic change, particularly in the 1970s. Indeed the drinks sales executive of International Publishing Corporation (I.P.C.) has concluded that, "the growth among women drinkers is the most significant factor affecting the drink market as a whole".'

(Shaw 1980: 10)

The types of beverages most commonly consumed by Scottish women in the past two decades have been wines and spirits. Among their counterparts in England and Wales, beer has been a far more popular drink (Wilson 1980a). The market for vermouths changed dramatically between 1969 and 1977. Between 1969/70 and 1976/77, the number of women who consumed these drinks rose by 140 per cent (Ratcliffe 1979). In 1978, when Ratcliffe's survey was undertaken, 63 per cent of all products in the vermouth market were being consumed by women. With the help of transnational corporations and their very able marketing research, a new range of drinks, the cream liqueurs, has been produced and aimed primarily at women (Cavenagh 1983). The new, stronger lagers have also become fashionable drinks for women. These are approximately two-and-a-half times stronger than ordinary lagers or beers. For this reason they are of more concern in relation to drinking and driving, for example.

It is clear that the alcohol producers feel there are great possibilities to encourage and channel women's purchasing power.

Society's view of women as drinkers has ceased to be one of overwhelming condemnation. Indeed, a brief examination of women's magazines shows how extensively the alcohol industry advertises in them. One advertisement for a vodka, for example, shows a woman in a carefree and provocative pose. The suggestion is that she owes her new-found liberation to the drink.

The owners and managers of public houses, too, are aware of this group. Grant has noted: 'Since too the beverage choices of women are different from the traditional male drinks, the effect is often to increase the aura of sophistication conveyed by the modern pub' (Grant 1982: 172). Dight conducted a general population survey of Scottish drinking habits in 1972. This study indicated that 46 per cent of women aged 17 and over were 'regular drinkers'. These were respondents who had drunk alcohol in the past seven days, most of whom reported that this was typical. The average amount of alcohol these women had consumed during the previous week was 4.8 units. Only six years later, a second survey of the general adult population in Scotland showed that women who were regular drinkers had consumed an average of 6.2 units during the previous week. The average previous week's consumption of Scottish women had apparently increased slightly.

(Each unit is equivalent to a single glass (half-pint) of ordinary beer, lager or cider, to a single measure of spirits or to a single glass of wine. Each of these units contains roughly 1.0 centilitre or 7.9 grammes of absolute alcohol. The normal Scottish measure of spirits is 1/5 gill. The equivalent spirits measure in England and Wales is 1/6 gill. That in Northern Ireland is 1/4 gill. Some 'special' lagers contain 2.2 units in a half-pint. There is no standard measure for wine. This definition is employed throughout this thesis.)

One of the more ominous developments has been the increase in alcohol consumption of young females. A study of alcohol use among teenagers in Glasgow by Davies and Stacey in 1972 concluded that 15 per cent of the 14-year-old female respondents reported never having drunk alcohol. A more recent study of secondary school pupils carried out in five schools in the Lothian Region of Scotland concluded that only 2 per cent of either sex reported never having tasted alcohol. This study provided the following comment: '32 per cent of the girls were classified as regular drinkers. . . . The average level of consumption on the last drinking occasion was 4.1 units' (Plant 1982: 92–3). The gulf between these findings may be in part attributable to the fact that the surveys were conducted in different locations and among respondents of slightly different ages. Even so, they are consistent with evidence (e.g. Dight 1976; Wilson 1980a, b) that the abstainer is becoming rarer in Scotland. Examining the relevant data on young females, it is possible to see an increasing number of this group who are certainly drinking more than females in the past, and are at the beginning of their 'childbearing' years.

Female alcohol use and misuse have clearly been increasing.

However, per capita alcohol consumption in the United Kingdom was about 10 per cent higher in 1900 than it was in 1979. Between these dates consumption declined to its twentieth-century low point during the 1930s. Since then it has risen dramatically and has virtually doubled between 1950 and 1980. These changes are illustrated in *Figure 1*. UK alcohol consumption has recently declined slightly due to the recession.

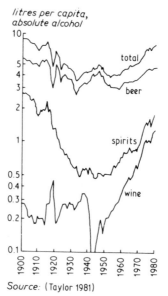

Source: (Taylor 1981)

Figure 1   Alcohol consumption by type, United Kingdom (1900–79)

WOMEN'S CHANGING WORLD

The role and status of women have been through a major and complex transition. Increased alcohol use and misuse are only a very small part of this metamorphosis. Young women are generally more confident and economically autonomous than were their forebears. The literature about female drinking contains many such phrases as 'the ransom of emancipation'. Whether this is interpreted as scare tactics or not, it is overly simplistic. Women are now more willing to question the acts and pronouncements of experts. The field of obstetrics is a good example. Some women are quite well informed about pregnancy. Many are more willing than before to accept responsibility for their own bodies. This has led to a reduction in the power that these women give to the relevant professional groups. It would not be possible for modern obstetric texts to declare: 'She [woman] has a head almost too small for intellect, but just big enough for love', as one did in 1848 (Shryock 1966: 184).

A large number of books about pregnancy have now been written by women. Kitzinger, for example, has written eight books on pregnancy and childbirth (Kitzinger 1962, 1977a, b, 1978, 1979a, b, c, 1980, 1981). Many others are also available (Oakley 1972, 1979, 1980, 1981; Hann 1982; Wright 1964, 1978). It is doubtful whether the editor of the *British Medical Journal* in 1984 would be wise to publish observations such as: 'If I were to plan with malicious hate the greatest curse I could conceive for women . . . I would estrange them from the protection of men', which the *Buffalo Medical Journal* did in 1871. The need to see men as protectors has been changing ever since Dr Marie Stopes opened her first controversial birth control clinic in 1921. The expanding number of self-help groups available today (ranging from women's consciousness-raising groups to pressure groups such as the National Childbirth Trust and Birthright) makes it clear that this trend continues. Presumably, few obstetricians in Britain today would give this advice to a new mother: 'have as domestic a life as possible . . . have but two hours intellectual life a day and never touch pen, brush or pencil as long as you live'. This guidance was provided in 1885, by Dr S. Weir Mitchell, a leading American physician.

The medical appliance manufacturers in the western world clearly see women as making more decisions about such things as positions in labour, for example. At a Women and Health Conference in Edinburgh (May 1983), there were no fewer than five different types of 'birthing chair' on display. The manufacturers seem in no doubt about either the intellectual or decision-making abilities of women, or their purchasing power.

FETAL HARM

Throughout the centuries the belief that parental drinking might cause *in utero* damage has persistently recurred. In ancient Carthage and Sparta, there were laws forbidding newly married couples the use of alcohol, in order to prevent conception while intoxicated. The Old Testament cites an angel talking to Samson's mother: 'Behold now thou art barren and bearest not; but thou shalt conceive and bear a son. Now therefore beware I pray thee and drink not wine nor strong drink' (Judges 13: 3). In his book *Anatomy of Melancholy*

(1621), Burton quotes Plutarch as saying, 'One drunkard begets another'. Whether he was describing genetics, social deprivation, or in utero damage is unclear.

At the beginning of the eighteenth century, Britain had an infant mortality rate that exceeded the birth rate. In 1726, the College of Physicians set up a committee to investigate the effects of alcohol consumption on the fetus. They traced mothers and fathers who were heavy drinkers and examined their offspring. They stated that parental drinking was 'a great and growing Evil which was, too often, a cause of weak, feeble and distempered children, who must be instead of an Advantage and Strength, a charge to their Country'. In 1834 a select committee of the House of Commons declared: 'Infants born to alcoholic mothers sometimes have a starved, shrivelled and imperfect look.'

However, the historical progression does not go unchallenged. Sir Francis Galton in his book, *National Interitance*, asserted the following:

'For example, a woman who was sober becomes a drunkard. Her children born during the period of her sobriety are said to be quite healthy; her subsequent children are said to be neurotic. The objections to accepting this as a valid instance in point are many. The woman's tissues must have been drenched with alcohol, and the unborn infant alcoholised during all its existence in that state. The quality of the mother's milk would be bad. The surroundings of a home under the charge of a drunken woman would be prejudicial to the health of a growing child. No wonder it became neurotic.'

(Galton 1889)

One of the first and best pieces of early research was reported by Dr William Sullivan in 1899. At that time he was deputy medical officer of a women's prison in Liverpool. He later became governor of Bedlam. The study carried out by Sullivan is described in more detail in chapter 1 of this book.

At this point, interest in the topic waned in both Britain and America. This was partly due to the Temperance reforms in both countries leading to the extremes of Prohibition in the United States. The world situation also changed both priorities and alcohol consumption levels, as illustrated by *Figure 1*. In 1942 the classic book, *Alcohol Explored*, by Haggard and Jellinek, was published. In this, the authors discussed the increased incidence of perinatal morbidity and mortality. However, they attributed these trends to poor nutrition and disturbed early home life. They concluded: 'The explanation is to be found in the fact that while alcohol does not make bad stock, the offspring inherit the defects of the parents.' In this way, the authors attributed the damaging effects of alcohol to genetic, social, and personal disturbances.

Concern about the possible ill effects of alcohol on the fetus was revived in the 1960s in France (see chapter 1), but it was in 1973 that Dr Kenneth Jones and his colleagues coined the phrase the 'Fetal Alcohol Syndrome'. These authors reported that:

'Eight unrelated children of three different ethnic groups, all born to mothers who were chronic alcoholics, have a similar pattern of cranio-facial, limb and cardio-vascular defects associated with prenatal-onset growth deficiency and developmental delay. This seems to be the first reported association between maternal alcoholism and aberrant morphogenesis in the offspring.'

(Jones *et al.* 1973: 1267)

It is possible to take issue with the last sentence. Even so, it is true to say that this paper in the *Lancet* led to a tremendous upsurge of concern and has generated a considerable amount of activity and literature. Most of the activity and writing has taken place in North America. Very little work in this field has been conducted in the United Kingdom. In addition, several key issues appear to remain unresolved and these gave rise to the present study.

1 Alcohol and the fetus: the background

This chapter presents a review of the literature related to the possible effects upon the fetus of alcohol consumption during pregnancy. This review relates only to evidence about pregnancy in humans. Animal studies are not comprehensively appraised, but the scope and implications of such work are briefly discussed. There is a wealth of material available on the topic – much of it tenuously linked to evidence of specific individual cases. This includes folk beliefs, speculations, political statements, and anecdotes.

For the purpose of this review, the evidence considered is divided into the following categories.
(1) Historical and general literature.
(2) Retrospective studies: clinical impressions and other relevant contributions to the literature.
(3) Prospective studies.
(4) Animal studies.

HISTORICAL AND GENERAL LITERATURE

The belief that alcohol can damage the fetus has been voiced periodically since the time of ancient Carthage and Sparta. As noted in the Introduction, in these cities the consumption of alcohol was forbidden by law to all male and female newly weds below the age of thirty, in order that 'defective children might not be conceived' (Haggard 1942: 210). The Roman God of Fire, Vulcan, was reputedly deformed at conception by his mother's alcohol intoxication (Heine 1981: 75) and Plato stated clearly his views: 'Children shouldn't be made in bodies saturated with drunkenness' (Burton 1906: 26).

Through the ages statements have been made in famous works. In the Old Testament an angel advises Samson's mother 'thou shalt conceive and bear a son. Now therefore beware, I pray thee and drink not wine nor strong drink and eat not any unclean thing' (Judges 13: 3-4). Feldman quotes a folktale from the Talmud that places responsibility squarely on the father's shoulders. 'Rabbi Nachman claims that his daughters are beautiful because he is an abstainer but Rabbi Bibi's daughter needs cosmetics because her father is "a drinker" ' (1927: 121-24). Tredrea also quotes the Talmud's warning: 'One who drinks intoxicating liquor will have ungainly children' (1983: 4). These admonitions are particularly striking since twentieth-century Jewish people have very low rates of alcohol-related problems (Snyder 1957, 1962; Davies and Walsh 1983). In 1621 Burton (republished 1906) in his *Anatomy of Melancholy* quotes Gellius: 'if a drunken man gets a child it will never likely have a good brain', and Aristotle: 'Foolish, drunken or hare-brained women [for the] most part bring forth children like unto themselves, morosos et languidos'.

In 1725 James Sedgewick, an English apothecary gave the following warning:

'half the train of chronical Diseases with which we see Children afflicted, are only the secondary Sighs, and Groanings, the evidential Marks, and Reproaches, of parentive ill-spent life. . . . These consequences may, nay without doubt, will be brought on Infants, by the Debauchery of the Mother . . . so that from the whole, the Regulation of the Mother, during her Pregnancy, is an Affair of the highest Moment and Consideration.'

(Warner and Rosett 1975: 1396)

A year later, in 1726, the College of Physicians in Britain petitioned Parliament to control the distilling trade, saying 'Parental drinking is a cause of weak, feeble and distempered children'. It is interesting to note that although different groups were agreed on the damage to the fetus, they were not agreed on the parent responsible. Plato, Aristotle, Gellius, the Old Testament, and Sedgewick are clear it is the mother's drinking that causes the damage, while the Talmud cites the father. Plutarch, the rulers of Carthage and Sparta, and the British College of Physicians are less specific. They indicate that both parents are responsible. This debate remains unresolved.

In 1775, for the second time, the British government set about controlling the retailing and taxing of gin. This was in response to pressure from groups such as the Committee of the Middlesex Sessions, as well as from vocal individuals. Perhaps the two most famous of these individual lobbyists were the novelist Henry Fielding and the artist William Hogarth. Henry Fielding, brother of the Parliamentarian Sir John Fielding, whose awareness of deprivation led him to try to set up one of the first police forces in Britain, queries: 'What must become of an infant who is conceived in Gin? With the poisonous Distillations of which it is nourished both in the Womb and at the Breast' (Warner and Rosett 1975: 1395). William Hogarth presented his concerns in more graphic form with his celebrated etchings, Beer Street and Gin Lane. He was one of the first people to actually draw the description of the facial features. 'Gin Lane' shows a baby falling out of the mother's arms; its facial features are different from those of the other children in the picture. In the words of the Committee of the Middlesex Sessions, it looks 'shrivel'd and old as though . . . numbered many years' (Coffey 1966: 671). These prints were widely distributed, perhaps in an early attempt at health education. The British mortality rate at that time, 1720–50, particularly of children under five years of age, was greater than the birth rate. As Morris rather confusingly attributes it: 'The present increasing diminution of the christenings in London beneath the burials, with many other evils [is due] to the enormous use of spirituous liquors' (Morris 1751: 89).

Eighteenth-century popular opinion did not object to alcohol *per se*, but to gin and other 'spirituous liquors' in particular. In fact, beer was widely held to be beneficial, a view that still lingers today. Most eighteenth-century obstetricians certainly would not have wished alcohol to be prohibited. They used it frequently as a drug and often gave very mixed messages because of this. Warner and Rosett quote Edward Foster, a Dublin midwifery professor, who stated in 1781 'that uterine haemorrhage leading to miscarriage or abortion could result from "the abuse of stimulants, vinous and other strong liquors" but recommended alcohol as a pain killer during pregnancy and delivery'. The nickname for gin, 'Mother's Ruin', appeared at this time. This folktale method of inducing an abortion with a 'hot bath and a bottle of gin' is still known today.

Benjamin Rush, a famous figure in American medical history and one of the signatories of the Declaration of Independence wrote an *Enquiry into the Effects of Spirituous Liquors upon the Human Body* (Rush 1787). Rush warns against alcohol being given to pregnant women, but his warning had little to do with the health of the fetus. His concern was for the woman, because of alcohol's potential for creating dependence. It was a widely held belief during the nineteenth century that any deterioration of the parental nervous system due to alcohol consumption could be transmitted directly to offspring.

Thomas Trotter first published his book *An Essay, Medical, Philosophical and Chemical on Drunkenness* in 1813 (republished 1981: 86–7). He warned women about misuse of alcohol on two counts. First, their risk of spontaneous human combustion, a strange phenomenon whereby people burst into flame for no apparent reason (see also Harrison 1977). Second, he predicted 'irregular menstruation with all its evils, and abortion in the early months of pregnancy, are the frequent consequences of inebriation in the fair sex'. He goes on to say

'can it be too gross to suppose, that the organs of generation must equally suffer in both sexes, from frequent intoxication: and if offspring should unfortunately be derived from such a parentage, can we doubt that it must be diseased and puny in its corporeal parts; and beneath the standard of a rational being in its intellectual faculties?'

(1813 republished 1981: 133)

Other medical practitioners of the time also expressed their concern. In 1827 Dr Robert McNish of Glasgow wrote: 'The children of such persons [confirmed drunkards] are, in general, neither numerous nor healthy. . . . They are apt to be puny and emaciated, and more than ordinarily liable to inherit all the diseases of those from whom they are sprung' (Warner and Rosett 1975: 1400).

As noted in the Introduction, in 1834 a Select Committee of the House of Commons, set up to explore the problems of drunkenness, reported: 'Infants born to the alcoholic mothers have a starved; (see p. 6) shrivelled and imperfect look.' Even Charles Dickens commented on the problem in *Pickwick Papers* 'Betsy Martin, widow, one child and one eye . . . never had more than one eye, but knows her mother drank bottled stout and shouldn't wonder if that caused it' (1836: 191). The *Lancet* entered the debate in 1842 with a discussion between a Dr Clutterbuck and Dr Beaumont, who wrote: 'Females who abstain from alcoholic drinks enjoy, during pregnancy, an immunity from many distressing symptoms incident to this interesting period' (1841–42: 343).

Not surprisingly, these views were dependent to a large degree on the amount and pattern of alcohol consumption in the general population. Some opponents of heavy drinking and drunkenness, particularly the Temperance reformers, were prepared to accept that 'moderate drinking' was not harmful. Indeed, one of America's Temperance reformers, John Forbes, thought that alcohol might be advisable for pregnant and lactating women with digestive problems. In the 1870s Sir Ashley Cooper, a famous British court physician and surgeon, looked at the problem from a view other than that of physical damage, and he stipulated the problem-beverage type. He states 'The beer drinkers' children too were particularly prone to hereditary handicaps partly because beer has a certain anamalizing tendency' (Furnas 1965: 77).

Strangely, very few of these distinguished commentators seem to have examined, or even mentioned, the poly drug use that was prevalent throughout the eighteenth and nineteenth centuries. One of the most popular legal drugs in Britain at that time was opium. As Berridge and Edwards (1981) have noted 'Opium's inclusion with turnips and rhubarb in the agricultural discussions of the period was one sidelight on the content of agricultural innovation. It was an indication too of the drug's acceptability' (1981: 11). At the end of the eighteenth century, the Society of Arts and the Caledonian Horticultural Society actually gave prizes for the best crops of home-grown opium. The drug was an ingredient of everything from throat lozenges, to the well-known tincture of opium, laudanum. The use of opium was widespread in a way that is hard to appreciate from a modern perspective.

The misuse of opium and its derivatives certainly caused the political and medical figures of the time a great deal of concern. As Berridge and Edwards write:

'Self-medication with opium, if anything, encompassed more than the professional spectrum of use. A particular example was the connection of opium use with drinking. Certainly the conjunction of opium and alcohol in popular usage was more extensive than its orthodox use and it was popularly used to counteract the effect of too much drink. In many industrial working class areas, children's cordials containing opium were on sale in the pubs. . . . It is the custom for the publicans to keep a supply of laudanum to add to the brandy. . . . This appears to have been a widespread popular means of controlling and counteracting excessive drinking.'

(Berridge and Edwards 1981: 33)

Berridge and Edwards also describe the view of the medical profession that emerged: 'In 1892 the Inebriates Legislation Committee of the British Medical Association began for the first time to press for the inclusion within the Act of forms of intoxication other than the alcoholic form, [for instance] chloral opium and other varieties of habitual drunkenness' (1981: 166). This close connection between misuse of opium and alcohol is often missed. The description of the offspring of chronic opium users is strikingly similar to that associated with the fetal alcohol syndrome 'the poor, wizened, ill-nourished infants are really pitiable to behold' (1981: 104).

Another belief firmly held at this time was that the baby's health was governed by the mother's imagination. In his book, *Antenatal Pathology and Hygiene: The Embryo*, Ballantyne gave a fascinating review of the beliefs of the time. With allusion to the Greeks and Spartans and their laws, Ballantyne tells of the laws of Sparta that required wives to look upon statues or paintings of the strong and beautiful. This notion continued almost unabated for centuries. He stated, 'In the seventeenth century the attitude of the profession towards the doctrine of maternal impressions was one of blind credulity; but in the eighteenth this was quickly changed for one of sceptical criticism' (1904: 114). In Scotland, Munro, in his *Medical Essays and Observations* (1734) placed greater emphasis on the nutritional status of the fetus and completely discounted impressions made on the child by the mother's imagination.

However, the eighteenth century closed with faith in the importance of such impressions still strong. Geoffrey Saint Hilaire records in his *Histoire des Anomalies* that 'in the third year of the French Republic an infant was born with the representation of a Phrygian cap of liberty on the left breast, and to the mother the Government awarded the above sum (400 francs per annum), presumably for her patriotic thoughts!' (Ballantyne 1904: 119).

The second half of the eighteenth century witnessed the emergence of many new ideas in the form of English translations of European work. As Warner and Rosett so succinctly state: 'Benedict-Augustin Morel, known as a forefather of modern psychiatry, had coined an elaborate theory of degeneracy in 1857. Under Morel's system, parental drunkenness produced depravity, alcoholic excess, and degradation in the first generation of offspring, with progressively more severe symptoms in their children, until the fourth generation developed sterility, heralding the extinction of the line. Auguste-Henri Forel, another early psychiatrist, originated the theory that alcohol caused germ damage or "blastophthoria" ' (1975: 1403). In 1879 Long, in an attempt to quantify the problem, gathered information from medical practitioners in Michigan. His findings showed that in the opinion of these doctors, 21 per cent of inherited disease and 20–30 per cent of inherited 'degeneracy' could be attributable to alcohol. The key phrase in this study is 'in the opinion of these doctors'. However, there appears to have been no attempt at standardization of the criteria used to assess abnormality or to gauge the involvement of alcohol.

The National Society for the Prevention of Cruelty to Children was founded during the 1890s. Protection for babies and children had begun in earnest. Even so, it was still a number of years before protection of the fetus evoked similar concern. Interest in the subject of drinking in pregnancy and fetal harm waned during the beginning of the twentieth century. As noted in the Introduction, this certainly reflected the general decline in per capita alcohol consumption and the rise in the influence of the Temperance Movement, from which was emerging the Women's Movement. Alcohol consumption in the United Kingdom declined by over 50 per cent and Prohibition was introduced in the United States between 1919 and 1933.

However, the decline in interest in the possible effects of alcohol on the fetus was not total. During the first decade of the twentieth century a few papers were published by such people as Robinovitch, who divided 'infant alcoholics' into two groups. These were: 'hereditary (congenital) who were weak, likely to die in infancy' and 'acquired who developed problems due to the passing of alcohol from the mother in the breast milk' (Warner and Rosett 1975: 1407).

The advent of Prohibition in America understandably led to a temporary loss of interest in this particular alcohol-related problem. Strangely, Britain also seemed to share this loss of interest in the topic. In contrast, widespread medical interest in the damaging effects of alcohol in adults and the concept of 'alcoholism' as a disease prevailed. Discussion at this time suffered from the dismissive way in which it treated much of the previous Temperance literature. In spite of the often judgemental and moralistic overtones of the writers of the early part of this century, some Temperance writers still had valid comments to make. The risk of dismissing these was almost literally one of throwing the baby out with the bath water.

The first volume of the *Quarterly Journal of Studies on Alcohol* (now the *Journal of Studies on Alcohol*) included a paper by Jellinek and Jolliffe that stated: 'In spite of the practically unanimous opinion that the idea of germ poisoning by alcohol in humans may be safely dismissed, the spook of Forel's blastophthoria is still haunting German journals' (1940: 162). It is unclear where the 'practically unanimous opinion' originated. Haggard and Jellinek, in their book *Alcohol Explored* (1942), voiced a forthright view of the possible implications of alcohol misuse at conception: 'The belief that intoxication at the time of procreation might cause damage to the child . . . has maintained itself up to present times. . . . On the basis of present knowledge, however, it may be dismissed' (1942: 205).

No supporting information was provided about the 'present knowledge' and from where this evidence stemmed remains a mystery. Jellinek and Haggard go on to state: 'The fact is that no acceptable evidence has ever been offered to show that acute alcoholic intoxication has any effect whatsoever on the human germ, or has any influence in altering heredity, or is the cause of any abnormality in the child' (1942: 207). They do not, however, clarify why available evidence is, in their view, unacceptable. They identified two factors that they thought might mislead one to assume that alcohol might harm the fetus. The first of these was the poor nutritional status of some heavy-drinking mothers in pregnancy. The second factor was the damaging influence of a deprived, disturbed home environment. These issues are certainly relevant and important. Even so, Jellinek and Haggard appear to have assumed that these factors are the only two reasons for fetal damage, rather than two of many contributing factors. Their view of the home environment as virtually the only relevant influence upon childhood development was beginning to become the 'fashionable', if sometimes grossly reductionist, explanation of all manner of ills.

Warner and Rosett quote part of a question and answer section in the *Journal of the American Medical Association* of 1942. They note that the journal:

'printed the query of a reader who asked if 36 ounces of beer taken by a pregnant woman would harm the fetus. The response stated that even large doses of alcohol had not been proved harmful to the human fetus, stressing that animal experiments correlating maternal alcoholism with miscarriages or congenital defects were not directly applicable to humans.'
(Warner and Rosett 1975: 1412)

This dismissal of the potentially damaging effects of alcohol on the fetus continued. In 1955, Keller, from the Rutgers Center for Alcohol Studies, wrote in a pamphlet: 'The old notions about children of drunken parents being born defective can be cast aside, together with the idea that alcohol can directly irritate and injure the sex glands' (1955: 10). While little scientific work was going on, the proponents of this view became more vociferous. As late as 1965 Ashley Montague in his book *Life Before Birth* asserted: 'It can now be stated categorically after hundreds of studies covering many years, that no matter how great the amounts of alcohol taken by the mother – or by the father for that matter – neither the germ cells nor the development of the child will be affected' (1965: 114).

In 1977 Kessel in Britain stated: 'From the public health point of view the evidence at the moment is not strong enough to justify any statement that women who drink *moderately* during pregnancy are harming their unborn children' (Kessel 1977: 89). Statements were becoming more careful about amounts of alcohol consumed.

The Royal College of Obstetricians and Gynaecologists Scientific Advisory and Pathology Committee declared in April 1983 that:

'We feel, therefore, that there is insufficient evidence available to support the abolition of alcohol during pregnancy, but that excessive drinking is related to adverse effects on fetal growth and development, and it is not known at what level drinking is said to be safe. Therefore, women should be aware of the possible detrimental effects of alcohol during pregnancy.'
(Tredrea 1983)

British Governments of whatever political orientation have been equally diffident towards this issue. In 1981 the Department of Health and Social Security publication *Drinking Sensibly* issued the following declaration: 'There is evidence that excessive drinking during pregnancy can damage the unborn child but the extent of the drinking necessary to cause such damage is such that it would be advisable on health grounds to reduce the intake greatly irrespective of pregnancy' (1981: 13). However, a press release in December 1983 stated:

'There is no doubt that heavy drinking, whether regular or occasional, can harm the foetus and should be avoided during pregnancy or when pregnancy is contemplated. . . . Expert opinion is divided as to the extent to which lighter alcohol intakes are harmful to the foetus and whether there is a threshold below which it is safe to drink, but there is no doubt that alcohol passes from the mother to the foetus. In one British investigation, an intake of 10 single drinks a week was associated with a significant increased risk of bearing a baby of low birthweight, which therefore starts life at a disadvantage. Drinking at, or above, this level when pregnancy is contemplated or during pregnancy should be avoided. Whether drinking at these levels has other effects on the foetus has not been established. Neither has it been established that lesser amounts are safe, and there does seem sense in keeping alcohol consumption as low as possible during pregnancy or when pregnancy is contemplated.'
(DHSS 1983: 1–2)

The Health Education Council for England and Wales have also stated: 'More and more doctors think it is wise to avoid alcohol during pregnancy. So if you are pregnant or planning a pregnancy, NEVER drink heavily or frequently, and certainly avoid binges. Best of all, stay off alcohol altogether until your baby is born' (HEC 1983: 9). The messages are clear but not threatening. Sadly, at the time of writing, the messages given by the Scottish Health Education Group are not clear. In their publication *Book of the Child*, given to each prospective mother in the antenatal clinic, they have a section headed drinking and smoking, which says: 'Don't'. The following two paragraphs then talk of the risks of smoking but do not mention reasons or risk associated with drinking during pregnancy.

In 1980 the National Council for Women in the United Kingdom published the findings of their Working Party on Alcohol Problems. In their conclusions and recommendations they state: 'We firmly believe, however, that women have a right to know of the risks they may be incurring' (1980: 17). They go on to say: 'In our view it is inexcusable to allow even one child to be born mentally or physically handicapped in the slightest degree, simply because its mother was not warned of the potential risk' (1980: 18).

The Royal College of Psychiatrists certainly has been impressed by the weight of accumulating evidence. Their advice has changed since 1979, when their Special Committee made the following public statement.

'There is no evidence that a mother who drinks moderate amounts of alcohol is going to do her baby any harm, but there is increasing evidence that a mother's heavy drinking can do damage to the fetus. What in this context is meant to be "moderate" as compared to heavy is, as ever, difficult to quantify precisely, but a local equivalent to say a couple of bottles of wine taken each day is getting into the danger area.'
(1979: 83)

A revised edition of the Report contained the following addendum:

'Recent scientific evidence suggests that the potential dangers of maternal drinking during pregnancy should be further emphasised. Even very moderate social drinking may be associated with decreased birth weight and an increased risk of spontaneous abortion. The precise level of alcohol intake which carries seriously enhanced risk of the child's developing the foetal alcohol syndrome still remains rather uncertain. . . . In the light of this evidence the College would wish to recommend that women be well advised not to drink alcohol during pregnancy. . . . This advice supersedes the previous statement on drinking during pregnancy.'
(Royal College of Psychiatrists 1982: 69)

The United States Surgeon General (1981) is also very clear:

'Even if she does not bear a child with full FAS, a woman who drinks heavily is more likely to bear a child with one or more of the birth defects included in the syndrome. Microcephaly, which is associated with mental impairment, is one of the more common of these defects. Each patient should be told about the risk of alcohol consumption during pregnancy and advised to not drink alcoholic beverages and to be aware of the alcoholic content of foods and drugs.'

(United States Surgeon General 1981: 1)

On balance, the official response to this issue has been far greater in the United States than it has been in the United Kingdom. However, the question of whether the United States Surgeon General has moved too far too fast has been debated. As Kolata states:

'At the heart of the dispute over the no-drinking advice is the perennial question of how safe is safe. What kind of evidence is needed before a substance should be ruled harmful in any amount? Ruth Little, director of the alcoholism and drug abuse program at the University of Washington, asks: "What is the great benefit of drinking at all? That's what people should focus on rather than this frantic search for a safe level." On the other hand, Henry Rosett, director of the Fetal Alcohol Education Program at Boston University School of Medicine, says the government is losing credibility by crying wolf. "Doctors won't believe this advisory. They are skeptical of simplistic propaganda." '

(Kolata 1981: 642)

Both Little and Rosett were stating highly personal views on this issue. Both these are, of course, open to dispute. However, when the Surgeon General's statement was published, a growing body of evidence certainly justified some form of public acknowledgement of the possible dangers of even moderate drinking in pregnancy. In relation to many public health issues, recognition and concern may precede the accumulation of clear cut or persuasive evidence. It is possible, as Rosett asserted, that the Surgeon General's statement was rather more forthright than was justified by current evidence. However, in the light of the Thalidomide tragedy that America avoided, it was a reasonable response for the Surgeon General, or any other authority responsible for public health, to adopt a stance of caution, rather than one of complacency. Hindsight might prove this to have been extreme. That is infinitely preferable to ignoring or even perpetuating a potentially major risk.

Griffith Edwards, one of Britain's leading alcohol experts, aptly summed up the dilemma in his article for the *British Medical Journal* in 1983. He wrote:

'Alcohol problems notoriously attract absolutism, and covert moral stances easily become confused with medical advice. Threats to the unborn child excite particular anxiety. Lobbyists may seize on such an issue to manipulate support for a cause. Whatever the real biological problem, the story of the fetal alcohol syndrome might also profitably be studied in terms of what the sociologists would call the "social construction" of a problem. But with all those provisos duly entered, the Surgeon General and the Royal College of Psychiatrists are giving no more than responsible and tempered public health advice which does not outrun the evidence: the premise is not that moderate drinking carries proved dangers to the fetus but only that the possibility of such dangers have to be entertained. The individual doctor has the responsibility of deciding what he will say to the expectant mother about her drinking, but questions on drinking must now be included in routine prenatal assessment. The alcoholic woman who is pregnant most certainly needs urgent and compassionate help.'

(Edwards 1983: 248)

RETROSPECTIVE STUDIES

Most of the evidence in this field is retrospective. For the purpose of this review such material has been dichotomized into statements and publications that are primarily impressionistic or relate to a narrow data base. More substantial studies, including larger numbers of cases, or more rigorous or standardized data collection are described separately.

CLINICAL IMPRESSIONS

The difference between scientist and clinician is never more obvious than in relation to their orientations towards new research findings. As Rosett has commented:

'The basic scientist is tempted to wait until the definitive data are analysed before making recommendations. However, the clinician cannot wait, since patients request and need advice. Frequently, physicians must make recommendations based on their interpretations of incomplete information.'

(Rosett 1980: 119)

In many areas of health, clinical impressions not only precede, but often stimulate research. The fetal alcohol syndrome is an example of this. This section briefly reviews the impressions that have mainly been reported by paediatricians and obstetricians.

The fetal alcohol syndrome

As noted in the Introduction, Jones *et al.* (1973) coined the phrase the 'fetal alcohol syndrome'. The number of alleged cases of this reported syndrome in the literature snowballed. As Seixas points out in his paper 'Fetal Alcohol Syndrome and the Year of the Child':

'Further reports have been made from France (Hermier *et al.* 1976) and also from Germany where the cardiac anomalies have been particularly studied (Loser *et al.* 1975, 1976), Italy (Loiodice *et al.* 1975), Ireland (Barry and O'Nuallan 1975), the USSR (Skosyreva 1973; Shurygin 1974), Czechoslovakia (Zizka *et al.* 1978), Poland (Loiodice *et al.* 1978), Hungary (Koranyi and Csiky 1978; Pocsy and Balassa 1978), Japan (Okada 1978), Denmark (Rasmussen and Christensen 1978; Brandt and Miller 1978) and Spain (Cahuana *et al.* 1977; Garrido-Lestache 1976).'

(Seixas 1979: 323)

Majewski has published some relevant work on measuring levels of severity. In his study of 108 cases he classified alcohol embryopathy

Table 1   Some clinical reports of cases of the fetal alcohol syndrome

author	date	country	number of reported cases	features noted
Root *et al.*	1975			hypothalamic-pituitary function
Bierich *et al.*	1975	West Germany	24	usual features
Christoffel *et al.*	1975		One pair dizygotic twins	usual features
Olegard *et al.*	1975	Sweden	52	usual features
Goetzman *et al.*	1975	USA	3	usual features
Margolin	1977	USA	1	usual features
Hayden and Nelson	1978	South Africa	2	usual features
Qazi *et al.*	1979	USA		chromosomal and renal abnormalities
Hobbick *et al.*	1979		3	liver abnormalities
Steeg and Woolf	1979	USA		cardiovascular abnormalities
Mena *et al.*	1980	Chile	19	usual features
Smith *et al.*	1981	USA	76	usual features skeletal features
Dehaene *et al.*	1981	France	45	usual features
Iosub *et al.*	1981	USA	63	usual features
Halliday *et al.*	1982	Northern Ireland	23	usual features
Poskitt *et al.*	1982	England	5	usual features
Friedman	1982			neural tube defects
Qazi *et al.*	1982	USA	6	usual features
Beattie *et al.*	1983	Scotland	40	usual features

into three degrees of severity (1981: 129). Several other papers have been published that have reported babies identified as exhibiting features of the fetal alcohol syndrome. Some of these are summarized in *Table I*.
Due to the fact that investigations into this topic have now been going on since the late 1960s, there are papers presenting cases of older children. Fryns *et al.* (1977) described four fetal alcohol syndrome cases out of a systematic study of 500 institutionalized mentally retarded male individuals. Their ages ranged from 15 to 19 years of age. Streissguth *et al.* (1976) examined twelve fetal alcohol syndrome children ranging in age from 14 months to 4 years. Darby *et al.* (1981) followed up eight of these children ranging in age from 14 months to 6 years. Robe *et al.* (1979) discussed a delay in onset of menstruation among daughters of heavy drinkers. This particular study has many weak points but it did raise important issues and suggested lines of possible further work in this area.

Fetal alcohol effects

The Seattle study, which is discussed below, was in the forefront of scientific interest in the more subtle harm that may be caused by drinking during pregnancy. Other studies include Goodwin *et al.* (1975), Fox *et al.* (1978), Shaywitz *et al.* (1980), and Tennes and Blackard (1980). In addition, several studies have been related to placental transfer and elimination of alcohol, Seppala *et al.* (1971), Gartner and Ryden (1972), Idanpaan-Heikkilä *et al.* (1972), Waltman and Iniquez (1972), Mann *et al.* (1975), and Baldwin *et al.* (1982). The alcohol-acetaldehyde debate has been discussed by Kumar (1982). Interestingly, Veghelyi *et al.* (1978) have attempted to assess pregnant women who would be at risk of fetal damage by test dosing with alcohol and then checking acetaldehyde levels. Olsen *et al.* (1983) assessed alcohol use, conception time, and birth weight. Researchers have now investigated many aspects of the relationships between alcohol and pregnancy outcome and even considered topics such as alcohol's effect on the milk-ejecting reflex in lactating women (Cobo 1973).
Another perspective on this general topic is represented by several papers related to the obstetric use of alcohol as a treatment for premature labour (Lele 1982) and conversely, the use of alcohol to induce mid-trimester abortion (Gomel and Carpenter 1973). Other publications, while containing no original data, have provided useful reviews of the general topic, which have independently high-

lighted some key issues (Hanson 1977; Clarren and Smith 1978; Erb and Andresen 1978; Morrison and Maykut 1979; Chernoff 1980; Chernoff and Lyons Jones 1981; Woollam 1981; Furey 1982). What seems clear, is that increasing clinical awareness of the possibility of fetal harm due to drinking in pregnancy, also increases the number of children thus diagnosed. This does not mean that the numbers of the latter are necessarily increasing but rather that heightened awareness leads to recognition.

The clinical reports noted above certainly indicate an upsurge of interest or acceptance of the possibility that alcohol consumption during pregnancy may cause birth abnormalities. This literature indicates that a substantial, impressive, and long-established body of opinion has noted a link between drinking during pregnancy and various types of fetal harm. While such data are historically important, they are overwhelmingly impressionistic and lack the persuasiveness of research that measures maternal alcohol consumption and that also takes due account of other possible causes of birth damage. A simple association between drinking during pregnancy and adverse fetal outcome is not enough. Such a link, if evident, may be attributable to a host of other factors such as social class, diet, other drug use, age, and past obstetric history.

OTHER RELEVANT CONTRIBUTIONS TO THE LITERATURE

One of the first reports of retrospective research into the association between alcohol consumption during pregnancy and fetal harm was carried out in Massachusetts by Samuel Howe in 1848. He examined institutionalized mental 'defectives'. He reviewed the family histories of 300 of these 'idiots', and found 145 had parents who abused alcohol. Clearly, the possibility of finding accurate case reports on family drinking habits at that time was minimal. Presumably, the reports noting alcohol abuse would have been confined to the most extreme and notable cases. This problem still exists. In addition, Howe's report did not clarify whether the noted association was entirely attributable to the pharmacological effects of alcohol or could have been due to many other features, such as genetic make-up. In Switzerland, Bezzola re-opened the question of whether intoxication at the time of conception caused damage. He examined the birth records of children born between 1880 and 1890. This showed an increase in the number of 'idiots' born nine months after the wine festivals! His means of controlling for other relevant variables is unknown.

Sullivan, deputy medical superintendent of the Liverpool prison, referred to five other studies that were carried out about this time:

'alcoholic parentage was noted by Bourneville in 62 per cent of a series of 1,000 idiots examined by him; by Marro in 46 per cent of criminals; by Penta in 30 per cent of criminals; in the Swiss prisons for juvenile offenders in over 45 per cent of the inmates; by Mme Tarnowsky in 82 per cent of Russian prostitutes.'

(Sullivan 1899: 490)

The body of research grew. Warner and Rosett quote an impressive list: (Shuttleworth and Beach 1900; Robinovitch 1901; Crothers 1909; Gordon 1911; Davenport 1913; Gordon 1916; and Glueck 1918). They state:

'MacNicholl in 1905 surveyed the school children of New York City in one of the largest studies on alcohol as a cause of mental retardation ever attempted. He found that of 6,624 children of drinking parents, 53 per cent were "dullards", whereas among the 13,523 children of abstainers studied only 10 per cent were *dullards*.'

(Warner and Rosett 1975: 1405)

This is an example of the seriousness with which attempts were mounted in the early part of this century, to assess the relationship of drinking in pregnancy to fetal harm.

In Edinburgh at this time, Dr J. W. Ballantyne, a world-renowned authority on obstetrics, and one of the primary movers in the establishment of antenatal care, summarized the evidence of Dr Duncan, a member of the Edinburgh Obstetrical Society and of Dr W. Sullivan in the following way.

'It must, then, be concluded that parental, and especially maternal, alcoholism of the kind to which the name of chronic drunkenness or persistent soaking is applied is the source of both ante-natal and post-natal mortality. It acts in all the three ways in which I indicated that ante-natal causes can be shown to act in relation to the increase of infantile mortality – *viz.*, by causing abortions, by predisposing to premature labours, and by weakening the infant by disease or deformity, so that it more readily succumbs to ordinary morbid influences at and after birth. By causing diseases of the kidneys and of the placenta, it also leads to that failure of the filter to which I have already referred; the placenta being damaged, not only does the alcohol more readily pass through it itself, but it is also possible for other poisons, germs, and toxines, to cross over into the foetal economy. So it comes about that the most disastrous consequences are entailed upon the unborn infant in connection with syphilis, lead-poisoning, fevers, and the like in the intemperate mother.'

(Ballantyne 1904: 64–5)

Another important British study was reported in 1910 by Elderton and Pearson who examined schoolchildren in Edinburgh and Manchester. This study caused great debate when it concluded that: 'no marked relation has been found between the intelligence, physique or disease of the offspring and parental alcoholism in any of the categories investigated. On the whole the balance turns as often in favour of the alcoholic as of the non-alcoholic parentage' (Elderton and Pearson 1910: 32). The opponents of these conclusions were highly sceptical, and indeed, a lengthy criticism was written by the celebrated economist J. M. Keynes, a member of the Royal Statistical Society, in that Society's journal. He stated:

'(1) The prenatal influence on offspring of alcoholic habits in the parents. (2) The postnatal and environmental influence of alcoholic homes. (3) The influence of hereditary characteristics commonly associated with, but not caused by, alcoholic habits. . . . The following are, I think, the conclusions at which we ought to arrive. With regard to problems (1) and (3), there is no evidence which justifies us in holding any decided opinion. With regard to problem (2), a large mass of general experience makes it exceedingly probable, as Professor Pearson admits, apart from his Edinburgh investigation, that alcoholic homes exert in general an evil environmental influence upon children. To the solution of none of these problems does the nature of the Edinburgh data permit that any substantial contribution should be made. . . . The problems are, moreover, so complicated, and the effects of the three distinct influences so indistinguishable when we deal with instances in the mass, that they seem to invite the application of experimental rather than statistical methods.'

(Keynes 1910–11)

As noted earlier, interest in this subject declined during the early part of the twentieth century and only re-emerged in a few studies, such as that by Butler (1942). In the United States Butler conducted a retrospective study of a group of 1,438 mentally subnormal people and tried to trace the histories of problems in their family. He found that 21 per cent of the males and 23 per cent of the females had a family history of alcohol dependence.

Coincident with the increase in post-war alcohol consumption, scientific interest in the subject experienced a resurgence during the

1960s. Most of the relevant publications that appeared during this period were in foreign languages, such as Rouquette (1957) and Christiaens *et al.* (1960). In 1968 Lemoine *et al.*, from Nantes in France, reported the findings of a study involving 127 offspring of alcohol-dependent parents. The authors did not distinguish between maternal and paternal alcohol dependence but stated that these children had a specific cluster of features that suggested a common denominator. The average IQ of these children was seventy. The facial features were characteristic: short upturned nose, receding chin, deformed ears, sunken nasal bridge. So too were the overall growth markers, small height, low birth weight, slow growth, delayed psychomotor and language development, and hyperactivity.

Shortly after this, in 1969, Christy Ulleland, a paediatric resident in Seattle's Washington County Hospital, noted a group of infants in her care who, despite expert attention, did not seem to be thriving. She examined each baby's case notes and identified a common factor. All six children had mothers who had been diagnosed as alcoholic. This discovery alerted Ulleland to the possible hazards of drinking heavily in pregnancy. During the next few months she identified another ten, similarly affected children. Ulleland's initial findings were presented at a conference arranged by the American National Council on Alcoholism (Ulleland 1972). Her work came to the attention of two dysmorphologists at the University of Washington, David Smith and Kenneth Jones. This team of Ulleland, Smith and Jones then entered the search for a link between maternal drinking during pregnancy and fetal harm. Ulleland's pioneering role in this respect was very important and is often overlooked. Jones *et al.* published their initial paper in the *Lancet* in June 1973. The purpose of this publication was to: 'alert physicians and other health professionals to a pattern of altered morphogenesis and function in eight unrelated children who have in common mothers who were chronic alcoholics during pregnancy' (Jones *et al.* 1973: 1267). It was not until November of that year that Jones and Smith, adding another three cases and again writing in the *Lancet*, named the disorder the 'fetal alcohol syndrome'.

The list of abnormalities described by Jones and Smith are illustrated in *Figure 2*. This list was based on only eleven children. An impression of the features allegedly associated with the fetal alcohol syndrome is presented in *Figure 3*.

Performance	OCCURRENCE OF ABNORMALITIES	%	
		100	prenatal growth deficiency
		100	postnatal growth deficiency
		100	developmental delay
		100	short palpebral fissures
		91	microcephaly
		36	epicanthal folds
Craniofacies		64	mascilliary hypoplasia
		27	micrognathia
		18	cleft palate
Limbs		73	joint anomalies
		73	altered palmer crease pattern
		70	cardiac anomalies
Other		80	fine motor dysfunction
		36	anomalous external genitalia
		36	capillary hemangiomata

Figure 2   Pattern of malformation

Source: Jones and Smith (1975)

This paper by Jones and Smith has been widely fêted as a seminal work in this field. Beyond any doubt the authors accomplished an important feat in bringing the issue of drinking during pregnancy to a wide medical and scientific audience. Their naming of the new syndrome served as a catalyst for interest, acceptance, and research. However, the account related to eleven children only. Data about their mothers were limited and it is possible that other factors, such as illicit drug use or poor nutritional intake, were also related to the pattern of abnormalities observed. As Hingson (1982) has pointed out, it was a bold and possibly even a risky decision to identify alcohol as the key factor when naming this syndrome. At this time, the evidence upon which that decision was made was extremely limited. The issue of maternal undernutrition was addressed by Jones *et al.* (1973). They concluded:

'The prenatal growth deficiency was more profound in terms of linear growth than for weight growth. This is in contrast to studies of generalised maternal undernutrition and underweight for length and hence suggests that a factor other than nutritional deprivation alone was adversely affecting prenatal growth in these children.'

(Jones *et al.* 1973: 1270)

However acceptable this explanation may be, the fact remains that all the mothers in this original study were on welfare. The risk

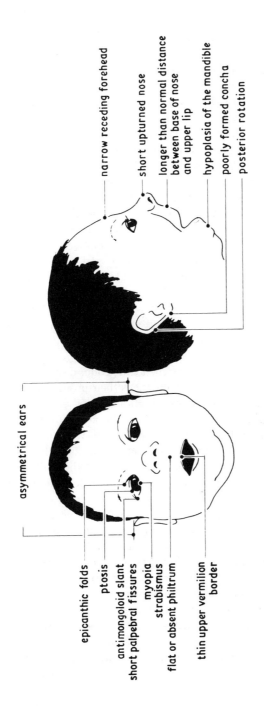

Figure 3 Features of the fetal alcohol syndrome

Source: Jones and Smith (1975)

category this puts them in cannot and should not be dismissed quite so readily.

The Seattle group of researchers proceeded to check through dysmorphology records and reported further observations of forty-one patients with the characteristic features of the fetal alcohol syndrome (Hanson *et al*. 1976). Streissguth (1976) then went on to report the intellectual development and motor performance of twelve offspring. All except one of the children were borderline or retarded in IQ. What seemed to be becoming clear was that the more severely physically disabled the infants were, the more severely mentally disabled they were. In addition, those with minor or more subtle physical damage, also had less easily detectable mental impairment. It must be kept in mind that at this point a lot of information was being collected on a relatively small number of children. What must also be acknowledged is that if the mother's drinking problem was even commented on in the child's records, then she must have been suffering from fairly serious alcohol-related problems. Then, as now, very few clinics take drinking histories in antenatal examinations. Only after the publication of these first few papers by this group did they become aware of the work of Lemoine *et al*. in France, which has been noted above.

The fact that these two independent groups described remarkably similar features certainly strengthens their position in terms of the persuasiveness of their observations. The Seattle group then attempted to use the data from the National Institute of Neurologic Disease and Stroke's Perinatal Project. This was a massive study on 55,000 women, beginning antenatally, continuing throughout pregnancy, and on for the first seven years of their offsprings' lives. Alcohol was not one of the initial topics included in the first interview, which is probably why only twenty-three cases of drinking problems were noted. Again, these would probably have been extreme cases. To prevent bias in producing assessments, the charts of the offspring were examined by fieldworkers who had no knowledge of the mother's drinking status. Each of these twenty-three were matched with two non-drinking controls on the basis of social class, age, marital status, and parity.

The results showed adverse outcome in 43 per cent of the alcohol misusing group, compared with only 2 per cent of the controls. Adverse outcome included perinatal mortality (17 per cent) and characteristics of the fetal alcohol syndrome (34 per cent). The methodology, in terms of the uncertain representativeness of the experimental group and the rather sweeping conclusions made on an obviously small number of cases, has been seriously questioned. Nevertheless, this was a large-scale controlled study and the differences between the experimental and control subjects were quite clear.

The Seattle researchers proceeded to organize a prospective study, in the hope of assessing more accurately the risk of fetal harm due to alcohol consumption in pregnancy. This study will be discussed in the following section of the chapter. In 1977 Russell conducted a retrospective study of intrauterine growth in women who were being seen for alcohol-related psychiatric problems. She hypothesized that women with these problems were more likely to have been drinking heavily during a prior pregnancy than women with non-alcohol-related problems. This is a rather improbable hypothesis, since present drinking patterns do not necessarily indicate either past or future drinking. Russel's findings, as summarized by Abel in his review of literature related to the fetal alcohol syndrome, were that these 'Offspring of women with alcohol-related problems weighed significantly less at birth. The longer the interval between onset of drinking and the birth of a child, the lower the birth weight; for every year of drinking there is a decrease of 24 gms in birth weight' (Abel 1981: 49). Although the birth weight measurement was probably reasonably accurate, the accuracy of alcohol-consumption histories was highly debatable, as stated earlier. Up to this stage, alcohol consumption was widely recorded in a rather vague or general way. This may have provided a good enough indication of the differences between individual women, it may or may not have been misleading. Nevertheless, alcohol-consumption patterns, being of crucial importance to this issue, warranted a more precise approach. Realistically at this point, it was evident that large-scale prospective studies were required.

This growth of concern was not confined to western countries. An International Populations Report on Rising Infant Mortality in the USSR in the 1970s contained the following statement:

'In November 1979 Kevin Klose of the *Washington Post*'s Moscow Bureau reported on a recent Soviet article showing a connection between rising infant mortality and a combination of female alcohol abuse and a high frequency of induced abortions. . . . This combination is present in 8 per cent of all births in Moscow, and the mortality rate of these infants is 30 times that of full-term infants.'

(US Department of Commerce 1980: 11. No further information is given.)

Gradually, the view that heavy drinking in pregnancy was fetotoxic became accepted, mainly in America. This charge was largely attributable to some prospective studies that are reviewed in the next section of this chapter. The next question was inevitable: what harm, if any, does moderate drinking in pregnancy cause?

In July 1980 the *Lancet* published a paper on the relationship between alcohol consumption during pregnancy and the incidence of spontaneous abortion. The authors of the study, Kline *et al.*, also from America, selected as its subjects 616 women who aborted spontaneously, and, as a control group, 632 women who delivered after at least 28 weeks gestation. Within the limits of their retrospective design, the authors completed a well conducted study. They elicited data on drinking before and during pregnancy using a quantity-frequency approach. In addition they controlled for the more common of the potentially confounding variables such as diet, smoking, and other drugs. Their findings were clear: 'Our results imply that alcohol causes spontaneous abortion. . . . Drinking as little as twice a week, above the minimum dosage of one ounce of absolute alcohol, is probably enough to endanger the fetus' (Kline *et al.* 1980: 180). However, Kline *et al.* did not control for social class. And indeed, all the women taking part in this study were receiving public assistance, which clearly puts them in an at-risk group for many problems. It also appears that Kline and her colleagues repeated the study with private patients and did not find any obvious effect of moderate drinking on low birth weight. As also noted by Kolata 'The women who aborted were interviewed nearer to the beginning of their pregnancies and so may have been more likely to recall how much they drank' (1981: 643).

In Japan, Tanaka *et al.* carried out a study that was published in 1981. Data were obtained by sending questionnaires to 2,573 hospitals of 300 beds or over, and institutions for the mentally retarded. The information requested was about parental drinking of the mentally retarded inmates. Only twenty-six cases were collected, and although the mothers' alcohol consumption is stated as being an average of 110 mls of absolute alcohol daily throughout pregnancy, there is no information on how this amount was arrived at, except that: 'Data . . . on their mothers were sent to us by doctors, other professionals and social workers from all over Japan' (Tanaka *et al.* 1981: 305). The results of this study are weakened by the apparently low response rate obtained, and by the totally uncontrolled and unstandardized nature of the data produced. Nevertheless, this contribution is of value since it reinforced, from a different cultural setting, a consensus that had been growing in the west.

A second, larger study of 488 subjects in Connecticut was published in the same year. This exercise by Berkowitz was primarily on preterm delivery. Data were obtained by direct interview and from case notes. The author identifies some of the limitations to her study, but goes on to say: 'Alcohol consumption gained statistical significance for the first and second trimester with the addition of such controlling variables as marital status and socioeconomic class' (Berkowitz 1981: 90). Berkowitz classes alcohol consumption prior to the third trimester of pregnancy: 'as a significant risk factor in pre-term delivery' (1981: 81). A second paper by the same author reported in 1982 on the effects of tobacco, alcohol, coffee, and tea consumption. Berkowitz states: 'Heavy alcohol consumption (an average of two or more drinks per day) . . . was associated with an approximately three-fold risk of pre-term delivery' (Berkowitz 1982: 239). These were valuable contributions, which acknowledged that many factors may be influential, including not just one, but several measures of alcohol consumption. Even so, alcohol-consumption data were reported vaguely. Apparently, little attention was paid to the pattern of drinking, which might be an important and relevant factor. Berkowitz does, however, raise a practical point that has caused some heart searching in the medical profession: 'Since alcohol has been used therapeutically to stop premature labour, the results of the present study were unexpected' (1981: 90). This issue has already been noted in relation to clinical impressions.

The problems associated with the collection of retrospective data in this field are clear. First, the alcohol-consumption histories, if taken by interview after the pregnancy, will be of uncertain accuracy due to poor memory recall. Also, they may be distorted, depending on pregnancy outcome. Second, ability to assess other confounding variables, such as other psychoactive drug use is also reduced. Third, interpretation of consumption histories may be distorted, due to the possibility of bias. This can be controlled for if the staff examining the babies are not aware of the information about the use and misuse of alcohol and other factors collected from the mothers after delivery. This problem also needs to be overcome in relation to prospective studies.

A fourth possible limitation of retrospective research in this field relates to indications in case notes that a pregnant woman was or is a heavy drinker. Such comments are likely to relate only to extreme and atypically conspicuous individuals. These individuals are likely only to be detected due to their unusual, perhaps disruptive, behaviour.

Most of the retrospective studies cited above have been flawed by the fact that information about the use of alcohol and other substances, before and during pregnancy, was collected months after the behaviour occurred, and was generally rather vague. In addition, the range of data relating to events before and during pregnancy was restricted to the information collected at the time. Retrospective studies have been heavily reliant upon collating whatever data were already available by chance, and often for other purposes. As noted above, only in exceptional circumstances do such data relate to either alcohol or other drug use.

Retrospective studies, whether purely impressionistic or involving the standardized collection of data from large study groups, have produced a virtually unanimous consensus that there is an association between alcohol consumption during pregnancy and fetal harm. This consensus has emerged from an impressive number of studies conducted by clinicians and researchers in a wide range of cultural contexts. As noted above, retrospective research is, in some important respects, less robust than prospective research. In spite of this, many of the defects of any one study have been compensated for by the virtues of others. Retrospective work has made an immense contribution to the literature on possible fetal alcohol effects and has identified the issues that led to the execution of the present study. Retrospective studies in relation to this topic, and more generally, serve as an invaluable bridge between folklore and clinical impressions on the one hand, and prospective studies on the other.

PROSPECTIVE STUDIES

The studies in this section are arranged in chronological order of publication date. Finally, the four main, recent large-scale studies, all of them American, are reviewed.

The first important prospective study of this topic has been mentioned briefly above. This was the investigation carried out by Dr W. Sullivan in 1899. Sullivan took a different standpoint from his colleagues. He decided:

'to take as the end of investigation, not alcoholism in the ancestry of the degenerate, but degeneracy in the descendants of the alcoholic. It has seemed to me that an inquiry from this point of view into the history of the offspring of the female criminal alcoholic might not only be of interest as a contribution to the study of that particular social category, but might also furnish results applicable, with certain reservations, to the general question of the influence of parental alcoholism.'

(Sullivan 1899: 490)

The study sample was selected from the female population of a Liverpool prison. Sullivan controlled for the confounding variables thought to be appropriate at that time. These did not include social class, drug use, and diet, which have concerned recent researchers. Instead, Sullivan examined what to him were the obvious and appropriate ones for his population, namely syphilis and tubercular disease. He also eliminated 'the subjects of markedly neurotic type who, [had] specially early and violent cerebral reaction to alcohol' (Sullivan 1889: 48). The series consisted of 100 women, twenty of whom were able to give details of female relatives with drinking problems. These 120 women had produced 600 children between them. He examined the psychological and physical histories of his subjects, and stated:

'the special nervous localisation of the poison was very marked: thirty-one of the women had suffered from one or more attacks of alcoholic delirium while twenty-four others, without actual delirium, had occasional visual hallucinations. Suicidal impulses, disorders of cutaneous sensibility, cramp in the extremities, were noted in a considerable number of cases.'

(Sullivan 1899: 491)

Sullivan's research was conducted and documented in a strikingly 'modern' manner. Even so, his study group was highly deviant and atypical. He checked type of beverage alcohol reportedly consumed by his subjects. Unfortunately, there is no attempt at measuring levels or patterns of consumption. Sullivan used as a control group the 'sober' female members of their families. He also considered, surprisingly, two of the issues that remain the subject of debate and investigation today.

First, regarding the influence of length of maternal drinking history on the fetus, Sullivan stated: 'that we find a sensibly higher infant death-rate in cases where the maternal inebriety has developed at an early period' (1899: 494). Second, the influence of paternal drinking. He concluded: 'If this result were confirmed with adequate figures it would suggest that . . . the influence of maternal drunkenness is so predominant a force that the paternal factor is almost negligible' (1899: 494).

Sullivan's conclusions were as follows: 'The death-rate amongst the children of the inebriate mothers was nearly two and a half times that amongst the infants of sober women of the same stock' (1899: 495). Of the 600 children involved in this study 265 – 44.2 per cent – survived more than two years, while 335 – 55.8 per cent – were either stillborn or died under the age of two. Sullivan scrutinized the women who had 'been drunk' at the time of conception but had spent most of their pregnancy in enforced sobriety: that is, in prison. He acknowledged the disadvantage of the small number of cases in which he could accurately assess drunkenness at conception and stated: 'In seven cases the condition was noted, and in six of these cases the children died in convulsions in the first months of life; in the seventh case the child was still-born' (1899: 495).

Sullivan concluded:

'Maternal inebriety is a condition peculiarly unfavourable to the vitality and to the normal development of the offspring. Its gravity in this respect is considerably greater than that of paternal alcoholism. . . . It is hardly necessary to point out in conclusion the evidence which these observations furnish as to the social gravity of female inebriety, and the social profit in its removal. In suppressing the female drunkard, the community not only eliminates an element always individually useless and constantly liable to become individually noxious: it also prevents the procreation of children under the conditions most apt to render them subsequently, if they survive, a burden or a danger to society.'

(Sullivan 1899: 499)

Sullivan did not explain how he would 'suppress the female drunkard'! But this was by far the best study carried out into this topic for many years. For more than half a century, published work in this field consisted of animal studies, clinical impressions, and retrospective data.

Between 1963 and 1969, Kaminski *et al.* collected data at twelve maternity hospitals in Paris. The main aim of their investigation was: 'the study of the etiology of congenital malformations' (Kaminski 1978: 155). Data were collected on alcohol consumption before and during pregnancy. However, in some geographical areas information on 'aperitifs or digestifs' was not collected. The reasons for this curious omission are unclear. This anomaly is made even more unclear by Lamache's observations to the National Academie De Medicin a few years earlier: 'Aperitifs and liqueurs . . . were found to be fairly common, along with wine, as the basis of alcoholism in the urban areas' (Lamache 1967). Kaminski eventually excluded the areas with only partial alcohol consumption data from the analysis. The results indicated that: 'Women consuming alcoholic beverages in excess of 40 cl of wine per day have an increased risk,' and that: '(1) The risk of still birth is elevated, especially death from abruptio placentae; (2) mean birth weight is lower, and the risk of a small-for-dates infant is increased; (3) placental weight is also decreased' (Kaminski 1978: 162). Kaminski presented the profile of women who drank over 40 cl of wine daily: older, unmarried women, with high parity, no professional activity, and in addition, lower socioeconomic status. These women were also heavier in weight than average, smoked, had a history of bleeding in early pregnancy and a previous history of bearing low birth weight infants. Kaminski acknowledges that the cut-off point of 40 cl of wine a day that was adopted for the purposes of analysis was an arbitrary one but goes on to say: '(1) Below 40 cl, there is no difference in the three classes of consumption; outcome for abstainers is essentially the same as for the two other categories [1–20 and 21–40]; (2) Risks rise in the group consuming 41–60 cl and increase with increasing consumption' (Kaminski 1978: 157). She also examined the association between alcohol consumption and placental weight, something that does not seem to have been done before. She found a *negative* correlation between these two variables.

This study did control for factors such as age, marital status, tobacco use, bleeding in early pregnancy, previous pregnancy outcome, and previous history of small-for-dates babies. The exercise was not conducted specifically to investigate alcohol consumption in relation to pregnancy outcome. Even so, this was a competent and informative study.

Between 1969 and 1975 Hill *et al.* interviewed 231 pregnant women in Houston, Texas about their over-the-counter drug use. They included alcohol in their list of drugs, but the breakdown they adopted into abstainers, occasional, weekly, or daily drinkers was not clearly related to levels of alcohol consumption.

In 1974 Mau and Netter published the results of a West German prospective study of 5,200 pregnant women. Sadly, for so large and topical a study, the main shortcomings of prospective studies in this field were apparent. Only vague details of maternal alcohol consumption levels and drinking patterns were collected. The following vague system of categories of alcohol and coffee consumption were recorded: never, rarely or frequently, and even these do not seem to have been defined more exactly. Only 0.1 per cent of the study group put themselves in the 'frequent drinking' group. It is reasonable to assume that respondents may have avoided this classification. More important, as it is not defined, it is in any event meaningless.

In response to the paucity of self-acknowledged frequent drinkers, the authors were forced to adopt an extremely conservative form of dichotomy. A mere 4.8 per cent of their study group said they had drunk alcohol, 95.2 per cent said they had not. This appears remarkable in a relatively high-consumption country (Plant 1981: 82). The results of this investigation, according to Dr Kenneth Warren in his Critical Review of the Fetal Alcohol Syndrome were as follows:

'Women who drank coffee frequently (45.1 per cent) had underweight babies more often ($p < 0.05$), but had pregnancies of normal duration. Women who had consumed alcohol had pregnancies of under 260 days duration and more abortions, but no higher incidence of low birth weight infants. Malformations were not more frequent in either the coffee or alcohol consuming groups.'

(Warren 1976:9)

The conclusions of this study are gravely undermined by the inadequacy of its methodology. Not only were the alcohol-consumption data of unacceptable detail, the researchers failed to attempt to control for other factors (such as other forms of drug use, age, and social class) that might also have been associated with pregnancy outcome.

Kessel (1980) and Woolf conducted a prospective study in London. This was designed to detect excessive drinkers attending antenatal clinics. A study group of 1,871 women completed the 'CAGE' questionnaire (Mayfield *et al.* 1974). This instrument is designed to identify people who have severe alcohol-related problems. It does not attempt to measure alcohol consumption. On the basis of this method Kessel and Woolf concluded that 5 per cent of their study group were excessive drinkers. This 5 per cent were then interviewed about their patterns and levels of alcohol consumption. As noted by Abel (1982), few women with severe alcohol-related problems attend antenatal clinics. Moreover, even before Kessel and Woolf carried out their study, evidence showed that the key issue was not whether women with alcohol-related problems produced damaged babies. It was whether or not specific levels or patterns of alcohol consumption were associated with fetal harm. The CAGE questionnaire alone was an inappropriate instrument to employ in this context. The authors gave no hint that they recognized the incongruity or limitations of their approach. On the contrary, they advocated not further or more detailed research, but simply refuted the need for a formal screening test at antenatal clinics. Whether or not this screening test related to alcohol consumption or to serious alcohol-related problems was not clarified. The conduct of the study and the position of the main author did little to advance this field of enquiry or to raise the level of consciousness of United Kingdom Health Authorities in relation to this subject.

Hartwig *et al.* (1982) reported the results of a prospective study that they had conducted in Berlin. The study was primarily aimed at investigating drug use in pregnancy but had included alcohol. One distinctive feature of this study was that the women who were the project's respondents were given booklets to fill in from the third to the ninth month of pregnancy. This instrument elicited biographical data, plus information on drug use throughout the period. Apparently, this is the only study to have used information gathered over such a large part of the course of pregnancy – 28 weeks. The results indicated a much lower level of alcohol consumption during pregnancy than other comparable studies. The percentage of drinkers (no clear definition available) dropped from 64 per cent pre-pregnancy to 5 per cent in the last trimester. Here we find the second distinctive feature of this study, namely the conclusions they drew from the results – not that the women perhaps got tired filling in these questionnaires, but that 'the distinct decline of cigarette and alcohol consumption during gravidity may be interpreted in terms of successful health education and a good system of public health' (Hartwig *et al.* 1982: 54). This optimistic view is sadly at odds with the general effectiveness of alcohol education, which has been disappointing (Grant and Ritson 1983).

Halliday *et al.* in 1982 reported the outcome of pregnancy in twenty-three women problem drinkers in Northern Ireland. These subjects were selected in the following three ways: known by GP as problem drinker; smelling of alcohol at antenatal clinic; and admitted drinking heavily in the antenatal interview. Surprisingly, no attempt was made to determine accurately the levels or patterns of alcohol consumption. However, the results of this were clear cut:

'Twenty-one (91 per cent) of the babies were small-for-gestational age
and many had head circumference measurements below 5th centile. Ten
babies (44 per cent) had abnormal facies consistent with "the fetal alcohol
syndrome". . . . Most of the babies have shown delayed postnatal
growth and six of the ten who are aged over 1 year have delayed
development'.

(Halliday *et al*. 1982: 892)

This is one of the first recent United Kingdom studies related to the
fetal effects of maternal alcohol consumption during pregnancy. It is
worth noting that alcohol consumption among women in Northern
Ireland is generally much lower than among their counterparts in
Britain. In contrast, rates of alcohol-related problems in that
province are relatively high (Wilson 1980b; Davies 1982).

As the authors note, twenty-one of the twenty-three women were
heavy cigarette smokers. No information was provided on the use of
medicines, illicit drugs, diet, general health, or the living conditions
from which these women originated. This study group were clearly
hard core or extreme problem drinkers. No precise information
about drinking patterns was collected, nor was a control group
employed. In consequence, though these women produced a
severely abnormal group of babies, this study alone, while consistent with other information in this field, in terms of ratio 1:1000,
twenty-three damaged out of 24,000 babies born over the time of the
study, did not cast much light upon the role of alcohol as distinct
from numerous other possible factors upon such abnormalities.

In 1982 Davies *et al*. undertook one of the few British studies to be
published at the time of writing. The researchers invited women
attending an antenatal clinic in Leamington Spa to complete a
self-administered questionnaire. The data collected included biographical details, consumption of alcohol, and other drugs. Blood
was taken for Gamma-Glutamyl-Transpeptidase measure. However, maternal height was not included: this would have been useful in
assessing abnormalities in babies' length. The alcohol-consumption
history included questions on 'binge' drinking as well as more
regular consumption. Davies *et al*. noted 'no association between
alcohol consumption and the number of abortions (22), stillbirths
(7), multiple pregnancies (10), nor between gender, gestational age
and Apgar scores of the babies' (Davies *et al*. 1982: 940–41). 'There
was a trend, however, towards smaller birthweight and head
circumference in the babies whose mothers drank more than 20 ml
[just over 1 unit] alcohol daily' (Davies 1982: 942).

This was a much needed attempt to assess the size of the problem in the area. However, waiting for long periods of time in the antenatal clinic may well have led to discussion between respondents about the questionnaire. No attempt appears to have been made to check that responses in an uncontrolled situation may have been biased by collusion between respondents.

Davies' assumption, that using a self-administered questionnaire in which the alcohol consumption questions were mingled with a number of unrelated items would lead to greater accuracy, appears to be questionable (e.g. Plant and Miller 1977). This study was a useful contribution and served to stimulate and to inform debate in a country where, strangely, this was previously lacking.

In 1983 the results were published of a British study of twenty-five women who were interviewed during the fourth month of pregnancy (Black 1983). Little will be found in a sample this size. Her decision to disguise the purpose of the questionnaire (because of people's tendency to underestimate) is ethically questionable and unlikely to be valid (Plant and Miller 1977) but her recommendations on the role of the primary health care team could usefully be taken further.

Gibson *et al.* conducted an Australian study that involved 7,301 respondents. The aim of this exercise was to seek associations between maternal alcohol, tobacco, and cannabis use and such adverse pregnancy outcomes as intrauterine growth retardation, congenital abnormalities, and low Apgar scores. The levels of alcohol consumption reported by this study were low – 25.5 per cent abstainers and only 1.5 per cent drinking more than 39 gm per day (approx. 3 units). This study was mainly focused upon cannabis use. Even so, the authors made the following comment in relation to the role of alcohol: 'In general the study supports the more commonly accepted associations' (Gibson *et al.* 1983: 18).

The only large-scale British survey at the time of writing was undertaken by Murray-Lyon and his colleagues in London in 1980. Information about the drinking habits of the first two hundred women involved, appeared in a letter to the *Lancet* in 1980. They conclude in this letter 'From the preliminary data it seems that drinking in pregnancy does represent a significant problem, at least in this selected area of the United Kingdom' (Murray-Lyon *et al.* 1980).

This study used two means of collecting information, by self-administered questionnaire and by interview. First, the respondents were interviewed by the doctor at the antenatal booking-in clinic. This was mainly for drinking history. Each respondent was then asked to complete a second questionnaire on pre-pregnancy drinking. This also included the CAGE and a shortened version of the Michigan Alcoholism Screening Test (MAST) inventory. This second instrument was to be completed at home and returned to the clinic. No rationale is given for this dual mode of data collection. Perhaps it was selected due to lack of time in a busy clinic. However, it does seems strange in that information on pre-pregnancy drinking need not take very long to obtain. The wisdom of using medical staff as interviewers in this type of study is discussed in chapter 3. Blood tests including blood count and Gamma-Glutamyl-Transpeptidase were carried out on all 1,122 patients. The research team then studied all 900 white respondents and assessed their offspring for such features as low birth weight. Their results are as follows: 'Alcohol consumption of more than 100 ozs a week around the time of conception carries an increased risk of low birthweight in the child. This effect is much more impressive in women who also smoke' (Wright *et al*. 1983: 664). This study has already produced interesting information, as noted above. In addition, it has also generated data on such topics as screening for alcohol misuse (Barrison *et al*. 1982) and use of medical staff as interviewers (Barrison 1980). The study involves 4,000 women. The final results are not yet published but this is most certainly the largest study yet carried out in Britain.

Tennes and Blackard in Colorado in 1981 examined 278 mother-infant pairs. They interviewed these mothers on two occasions during pregnancy, and once after delivery. They elicited details of alcohol consumption levels and patterns of drinking during pregnancy. The respondents interviewed in this study group were divided into two groups, the first related to total consumption of absolute alcohol during the whole pregnancy and the second group related to total consumption of absolute alcohol during one trimester. These measures were averaged by dividing by the number of drinking days and then compared with pregnancy outcome. This measurement of total consumption is unusual and not particularly helpful as it makes comparison with other work difficult. Tennes and Blackard state: 'The study design was intended to maximise data about alcohol use rather than about cases of high consumption' (Tennes and Blackard 1980: 777). Given the emphasis placed on 'binge' drinking and resultant fetal damage this seems a strange omission.

The findings in this study were different from most others, since a dose-response relationship did not emerge between moderate alcohol consumption and decreased birth weight. The small sample size and the confusing way of describing average alcohol consumption make it difficult to draw any firm conclusions from these results. However, as Tennes and Blackard state: 'Moderate amounts of maternal alcohol consumption were found to have no effect upon birth weight and not to be related to an increased incidence of minor physical anomalies' (Tennes and Blackard 1980: 780).

The remaining studies reviewed in this chapter are the main large-scale studies in the field and they are all American. In 1979 Sokol *et al.* in Ohio carried out a prospective study based on medical records from 12,127 pregnancies. This study was not primarily related to alcohol consumption data. As Sokol states: 'the perinatal data collection program was not implemented specifically in support of a study of alcohol abuse, so some detailed variables – in particular, volume and pattern information for alcohol intake was not collected' (Sokol, Miller, and Reed 1980: 142).

The only respondents whose alcohol consumption was noted were, as in several retrospective studies, the extreme alcohol misusers. Most of these 204 respondents fell into the category of older, unmarried women with previous poor obstetric histories. Presumably, because of the degree of severity of the alcohol misusers among his study group, Sokol pays more attention to these and discusses at some length management implications of the alcohol misusers in labour. Sokol and his colleagues then proceeded to set up a project specifically to look at alcohol consumption in pregnancy. This was one of the four major National Institute for Alcohol Abuse and Alcoholism funded studies. The other three were Rosett *et al.* in Boston, Streissguth *et al.* in Seattle, and Kuzma *et al.* in Loma Linda, California.

In this recent study Sokol *et al.* interviewed 2,913 women, screening them for alcohol-related problems using the MAST. This method of screening is used to detect people who have ever experienced psychosocial disruption due to alcohol. The goals of this study, as stated by Sokol *et al.*, are:

'(1) to determine the incidence of "alcoholism" in unselected gravidas registering for antenatal care in a public hospital setting, (2) to quantify alcohol intake longitudinally during pregnancy in study patients and matched controls, (3) to relate alcohol diagnostic and volume/pattern

data to measures of neonatal outcome, (4) to examine abstinence
oriented therapy with respect to infant outcome, and (5) to examine
interactions with other antepartum risks, such as smoking and maternal
illness.'

(Sokol et al. 1981: 204)

The 2,913 women were divided into positive and negative MAST
responders. The initial information about this study showed the
following differences between the two groups.

'Positive MAST responders were found to be more likely to drink
alcohol, to drink greater volumes and to drink more frequently than
matched negative responders. They obtained a smaller proportion of
their alcohol intake from wine and were more likely to drink a
combination of beer, wine and/or liquor than the negative responders.
The positive responders significantly decreased their alcohol intake as
pregnancy progressed, while negative responders did not, suggesting the
possibility that abstinence oriented therapy may be helpful.'

(Sokol et al. 1981: 203)

The drinking patterns of the positive MAST responders will come
as no surprise. This continuing study, eventually expected to
include 8,000 subjects, may prove useful in terms of examining a
particular population, that is pregnant women whose lives have
been disrupted by alcohol. As long as this study is run in conjunction with other projects that will examine possible subtle effects on
the fetus of moderate drinking in pregnancy, it will be useful –
particularly in implementing and evaluating programmes to help
this 'at-risk' group of alcohol abusing women.

A number of offshoots of these two studies by Sokol *et al.* have
subsequently been published. They have been concerned with topics
such as zinc status in pregnant women (Flynn *et al.* 1981), infant
development (Golden *et al.* 1982), and beverage alcohol (Bottoms *et
al.* 1982). There are numerous other investigations involving a
variety of sample sizes (e.g. Silva *et al.* 1981; Landesman-Dwyer
1981). One of these is from Seattle, one from Boston, and two are
from California.

In the first Californian study by Harlap, Shiona, and Ramcharan
(1979, 1980) the respondents (32,019) were given a self-administered
questionnaire to complete. This covered such topics as contraceptive use, alcohol and tobacco use, and past medical and obstetric
history. Additional data on previous obstetric history and health in
this pregnancy were elicited from clinic case notes. In common with

a number of other studies (Hanson *et al.* 1976; Berkowitz 1981) this exercise was originally designed for another purpose: namely, to examine the relationship between birth control and reproductive outcome. For this reason, the alcohol-consumption histories concentrated on average daily intake.

There appears to have been no attempt to assess patterns of consumption or to quantify 'binge' drinking. Some confusion may have resulted from the following wording of a key question related to alcohol consumption: 'during the first three months of pregnancy'. This is rather vague. Many women in Britain calculate the progress of pregnancy from the time it is given medical confirmation. The number of heavy drinkers was low, only 2.9 per cent of this study group reported having consumed an average of more than one drink daily during the first trimester; 51.7 per cent reported abstaining; and 44.7 per cent had less than one drink daily.

The results showed that risks for first trimester abortion were not associated with alcohol consumption compared to non-drinkers. The risk of second trimester spontaneous abortion was doubled for women who had consumed one or two drinks daily. The relevant variables controlled for in the analysis of these results included age and marital status. In addition, another variable was considered, namely previous history of spontaneous abortion. This is an important point in trying to identify the primary factor associated with spontaneous abortion, as a history of previous abortions could affect the course of a subsequent pregnancy. However, the possibility of under-reporting is high. In a country where the estimated number of women of child-bearing age with drinking problems is about 8 per cent, Harlap *et al.*'s 2.9 per cent again probably makes up the most extreme cases.

The second Californian Study was initiated at Loma Linda University and Medical Centre in 1974. The aim of this project was:

'to determine whether complications of pregnancy or subtle manifestations of Fetal Alcohol Effects are related to alcohol intake during the pregnancy and, further, to elucidate to what extent any observed damaging effects of alcohol intake can be accounted for by other correlates of alcohol, e.g. smoking, poor nutrition, drug abuse and certain sociological factors.'

(Kuzma and Kissinger 1981: 211)

This was, therefore, one of the first studies designed to look at the relationship between alcohol consumption and fetal damage specifically. The sample was large – 12,406 women. However, many of these women were lost to follow-up. The respondents completed a self-administered questionnaire during their first prenatal visit. This instrument included information on drinking, smoking, and other health-related habits. These questions appeared to be mainly related to pre-pregnancy drinking. Information on drinking and smoking during pregnancy was elicited *after* delivery. Given the short-comings of retrospective data collection, the lost opportunity to measure consumption shortly after its occurrence is a weakness in a prospective study. Alcohol consumption was estimated by a modified version of Cahalan's volume variability index. The surviving offspring were all examined by specially trained nursing staff. Telephone interviews were carried out with the mothers, 1 and 5 months postnatally, to obtain details of their infants' progress, feeding, sleeping habits, and any alterations in maternal alcohol and tobacco consumption. The sample was divided into four subgroups: abstainers, 31.5 per cent of the study group; those who drank prior to but not during pregnancy, 17.4 per cent of the study group; those who stopped drinking during pregnancy, 11.4 per cent of the study group; those who drank at all times, 39.7 per cent of the study group.

The last subgroup was divided even further by daily alcohol intake into: light drinkers, below 1 oz absolute alcohol; moderate drinkers, between 1 and 1.99 ozs absolute alcohol; and heavy drinkers, who are described rather confusingly as 2.00 to 2.99 ozs or over 3.00 ozs (Kuzma and Kissinger 1981: 213). The results of this exercise showed that a large proportion of the study group used alcohol and smoked tobacco during pregnancy and, as has already been shown in much epidemiological research, there is a high corre-lation between alcohol consumption and smoking (e.g. Dight 1976). The younger women and those with higher incomes were less likely to reduce their levels of alcohol consumption or to abstain during pregnancy.

This study was among the first to try to assess the effects of different beverage type. As the results show, '[frequent] heavy beer drinking during pregnancy is related to decreased intra-uterine growth' (Kuzma and Sokol 1982: 396). However, the authors noted that these results 'should be interpreted cautiously since there are several alternative explanations for the findings' (Kuzma and Sokol 1982: 396). Among the alternative explanations was 'The possibility that beer drinkers differ demographically, socioeconomically, and/ or in medical/obstetric risk level from women who drink mainly wine or liquor' (Kuzma and Sokol 1982: 401). Interestingly, frequency of wine drinking was correlated with *increased* birthweight.

It is regrettable that such an otherwise well conducted and large-scale study was weakened by the failure to collect alcohol-consumption data prospectively. It is by no means certain that this was a major cause of bias. Even so, available evidence does indicate that self-reports are more likely to be full if related to recent, rather than to distant events (Midanik 1982).

The Boston Study began in 1974 with a pilot prospective investigation of 200 women (Ouellette 1976; Rosett *et al.* 1976). The researchers used Cahalan's volume variability index to assess alcohol consumption and also collected information on use of other drugs, including tobacco, and nutritional status.

The results showed: 'a statistically significant decrease in all growth parameters in infants of alcoholic mothers' (Ouellette 1976: 127). This initial investigation was followed by more ambitious ventures. Between February 1977 and October 1979, 1,690 women who delivered singletons were interviewed retrospectively after delivery by trained fieldworkers. The latter were all women and the interview was comprehensive, of 30 to 40 minutes duration, and covered such topics as alcohol consumption, smoking, drug use, nutrition, accidents and illnesses in pregnancy, as well as biographical data. The respondents in this study were a young, low-income group, 60 per cent of whom were black. For the purpose of data analysis, these respondents were divided into three groups according to their alcohol consumption: light: abstainers or less than 0.5 drinks daily; moderate: 0.5 to 1.49 drinks per day, or if 1.5 or more, never more than five on any occasion; heavy: 1.5 or more drinks daily with five or more on some occasions.

The findings suggest that these women were more likely to have drunk heavily prior to, rather than during, pregnancy. Heavy drinking was positively correlated with smoking and illicit drug use. The latter also decreased in pregnancy. Alpert summarized: 'These data indicate that women who drink heavily during their pregnancy are very different in a number of ways from women who do not' (Alpert 1981: 200). Since the inception of the study a mass of data has been collected and analysed. Such topics have been examined as: neonatal morphology (Rosett and Sander 1979); benefits of reduction in alcohol consumption in pregnancy (Rosett *et al.* 1980); specific drugs (Hingson *et al.* 1982; Morelock *et al.* 1982; Hingson 1983); treatment of problem drinkers (Rosett *et al.* 1977; Rosett *et al.* 1978; Rosett *et al.* 1983); patterns of alcohol use (Rosett *et al.*

1983; Weiner *et al.* 1983). An important merit of this study is its attempt to control for confounding factors. Some evidence from this study suggests drug use, particularly cannabis use, reported by 39 per cent of the study group, may be an important factor in the development of fetal damage. However, as with some of the previously described work, the respondents came in the main from a high-risk, low-income group, whose pregnancy outcome for these reasons would be expected to be poorer.

Work continued on the Seattle study after the initial contributions by Jones and Smith.

Hanson *et al.* (1976), upon consideration of the most frequent clinical findings in forty-one cases identified as exhibiting the fetal alcohol syndrome, advised abortion for the alcohol-dependent woman who becomes pregnant. This recommendation is in striking contrast to the lingering reluctance of so many British authorities to even concede the possibility that drinking during pregnancy might be harmful. Ruth Little then gathered information on the alcohol consumption of 800 women both before and during early pregnancy, to provide one of the first prospective descriptions of this population. She found: 'maternal alcohol use before pregnancy and in late pregnancy is significantly related to infant birth weight' (Little 1977: 1155).

This group was followed up by Landesman-Dwyer *et al.* (1981). They found, according to the original author: 'children of moderate drinking mothers had significantly poorer attending behavior at four years of age. . . . None of the mothers . . . had consumed an average of more than four drinks a day during pregnancy' (Little 1981: 165). The idea of more subtle damage in moderate drinking women was emerging.

The next step was the larger Pregnancy and Health Study. This investigation, in which a sample of 1,529 women was interviewed, took place between 1974 and 1975. The study spans seven years. The aims were:

'to assess alcohol use as accurately as possible in an unselected group of pregnant women, to assess other variables both prenatally and postnatally which might be associated with maternal alcohol use and infant development, and to study the relationship of maternal alcohol use to offspring health and development.'

(Streissguth *et al.* 1981: 223)

Streissguth goes on to say: 'The primary focus of this study was the evaluation of behavioral characteristics in neonates and infants which might reflect early indications of central nervous system dysfunction and which might be related to intra-uterine alcohol exposure' (Streissguth *et al.* 1981: 223). Here is the key to the uniqueness of this study. The focus is on behaviour and intelligence, not just of childen of heavy drinkers, but also children of moderate alcohol users.

The women in this investigation were interviewed when 5 months pregnant. Information elicited included alcohol consumption, quantified by Cahalan's volume variability-quantity-frequency index and Absolute Alcohol scores. Binge drinking was included in this way. Additional information that was elicited included other drug use, namely tobacco and caffeine and dietary habits. The interviewers collected information on most of these for pre-pregnancy and during pregnancy. However, smoking pre-pregnancy was not assessed. The profile of these women was different from that produced by Rosett and his colleagues. These were middle-class, caucasians, on average twenty-six years old, with at least fourteen years education. After delivery, two cohorts were followed up: 250 heavy drinkers, and 250 controls who were infrequent drinkers or abstainers.

Both mothers and children were interviewed and examined at the neonatal period, 8 months, 18 months, 4 years and planned at 7 years. The initial results of this exercise showed that after controlling for smoking and other variables

'smaller infant size (birth weight, length and head circumference); lower Apgar scores, poorer neonatal habituation; decreased sucking pressure; increased tremulousness and head-turns-to-left; decreased vigorous activity; and a higher frequency of minor dysmorphic characteristics combined with low birth weight and microcephaly.'

(Streissguth *et al.* 1981: 223)

In common with other major studies in this field, this one has produced many further observations: maternal alcohol dependence (Streissguth 1976; Little and Streissguth 1978; Little *et al.* 1980; Streissguth and Martin 1983), newborn conditioning (Martin *et al.* 1977, 1979; Landesman-Dwyer *et al.* 1978; Streissguth *et al.* 1982) as well as a number of papers on consumption measures (Streissguth *et al.* 1977; Barr *et al.* 1981), methodology and measurements (Streissguth *et al.* 1976; Lund 1976; Streissguth *et al.* 1978; Little *et al.* 1979; Herman *et al.* 1980; Barr *et al.* 1981).

Due to the time span of this study, the papers now being published are describing an important aspect of this prolific pregnancy and health programme (Streissguth 1977; Little *et al*. 1980, 1981; Little and Streissguth 1981, 1982) and how the community education programme can change the advice given by professionals (Little *et al*. 1983).

The respondents in this exercise were more representative than in most other studies. Ideally, the women could have been interviewed earlier in this pregnancy, to help accurate recall of pre-pregnancy alcohol consumption. Nonetheless, this study has been well conducted and the initial and continuing evidence produced has placed it in the forefront of recent work.

These are some of the many studies, large and small, that have been published over the past two decades. One thing is certain: with refinement in techniques and statistical analysis to help control for confounding variables, we are nearer than ever before to discovering the association between alcohol consumption in pregnancy and more subtle fetal harm. Many reviews and bibliographies have now been completed on this topic; amongst the best are the three volume set: *Fetal Alcohol Syndrome* by Ernest Abel and his latest bibliography, *Alcohol and Reproduction*. Another good review has been produced by Rosett and Weiner (1984).

ANIMAL STUDIES

A critical review of animal studies is beyond the competence of this author. However, a tentative and selective attempt is presented to indicate the scope and some of the implications of such research to the fetal alcohol syndrome. Among the first to use animals as a means of measuring the effects of alcohol on the fetus was C. F. Hodge (1903). This researcher spent two years examining the effects of alcohol on the fetal outcome in cocker spaniels (Warner and Rosett 1975: 1407). His findings were inconclusive. Experimentation on animals has continued with considerable debate as to its usefulness.

Tittmar points out:

'Factors that may affect animal experimentation have been divided into four groups, namely genetic factors, environmental factors, the interaction of genetic and environmental factors, and those pertaining to the experimental procedure. Alternatively, these factors may be considered as being major sources of variable errors, and may, more conveniently, be classified as those sources associated with the subjects . . . those with the treatment groups . . . and those arising from replications.'

(Tittmar 1982)

His clear statement is equally valid in relation to many of the studies using human subjects.

The usefulness of animal studies is clear in terms of the relative ease with which it is possible to control for variables such as nutrition, genetic factors, and use of other drugs. Animal experimentation also permits evaluation of effects in a shorter period of time than would be possible on humans. Researchers do appear to have duplicated all the fetal alcohol syndrome effects observed in human subjects and in this way are helping to clarify the role of alcohol as distinct from other confounding factors (Chernoff 1977).

Animal studies have duplicated the features of the fetal alcohol syndrome in a variety of species, including: mice (Nice 1912, 1917; Swanberg and Crumpacker 1977; Randall *et al.* 1981); rats (MacDowell and Vicari 1917; Pilstrom and Keissling 1967; Martin *et al.* 1977); guinea pigs (Stockard 1913, 1916, 1924; Papara-Nicholson and Telford 1957); rabbits (Cole and Davis 1914; Schwetz *et al.* 1978); and dogs (Ellis and Pick 1980). For a detailed description of these and other studies the reader is referred to reviews by Abel (1980, 1982), Randall and Noble (1980) and Riley and Lochry (1982).

Research on animals has also increased knowledge and aided understanding of the following issues. Rates of elimination of alcohol during pregnancy and lactation (Greizerstein *et al.* 1979); social behaviour (Ellis and Krisiak 1975; Martin *et al.* 1977; Riley *et al.* 1979); malnutrition (Fisher *et al.* 1982), the question of a close-response curve (Ellis, Pick and Sawyer 1977; Clarren and Bowden 1982); the mechanisms involved (Mukherjee and Hodges 1982); the debate on the role of acetaldehyde (O'Shea and Kaufmann 1979).

It has now been demonstrated repeatedly that alcohol given in a variety of ways to laboratory animals causes abortion or reabsorption of fetuses, with resultant reduction in litter sizes and fetal abnormalities. Dobbing and Sands remind us of one of the major problems of interpreting the relevance of animal research for humans: 'We know of no way of telling whether a day in the life of a rat is equivalent to a month in the life of a human and even if it be so at one period of life it is likely to be otherwise at another' (Dobbing and Sands 1979: 80). However, as Sokol says 'By focusing on issues of current clinical impact, the laboratory scientist may contribute to improved pregnancy outcome in humans' (Sokol 1982: 183).

CONCLUSIONS

There is now a wealth of anecdotal and impressionistic information available. Many prospective research projects have taken rather vague consumption data and some have not controlled for the influence of factors other than alcohol that may affect pregnancy outcome. It is apparent that many ventures in this field have been conducted by busy clinicians. The latter frequently did not take advantage of the current survey techniques that are available for collecting information on alcohol consumption.

There is probably no such thing as the perfect study in the field of alcohol-related problems. The alleged association between maternal drinking during pregnancy and fetal harm is a singularly difficult area in which to conduct research. First, it is problematic as the number of possibly relevant or confounding factors is almost unlimited. Second, even prospective studies are partly retrospective because unless they first locate and examine their subjects before pregnancy (as in animal studies) details of alcohol consumption and other factors at this crucial stage are generally vague and collected months later.

The striking thing about the literature reviewed in this chapter is that it has produced a nearly unanimous conclusion that alcohol consumption in pregnancy is associated with fetal harm. Even so, the widespread deduction that alcohol consumption in pregnancy *causes* fetal harm appears to be based upon very little concrete evidence. On tests such as multiple regression, showing the predictive power of alcohol, their findings are not conclusive. There is a lack of information about the possible ill effects of alcohol consumption among a 'normal' group of women, most of whom are likely to be moderate drinkers. It is in the light of this that the present study was implemented.

2 Aims, design, and method

This study was mounted to achieve one primary aim: to establish whether or not birth abnormalities are associated with self-reported rates of drinking by pregnant women.

If this association was established, two secondary aims would be pursued: (a) to ascertain at what levels of alcohol consumption birth damage of various types is evident, and (b) to investigate whether the features of alcohol-related birth damage do constitute a syndrome.

DESIGN

A prospective design was selected primarily because retrospective data related to alcohol consumption and other key variables are of questionable validity. A retrospective study would have enabled the inclusion of more damaged babies in the study group. Even so, women who had already given birth to such children might have extremely poor recollections of their drinking in pregnancy. In addition, the trauma of the birth of a damaged child might have influenced perceptions and patterns of response. Accordingly, it was decided to adopt a prospective design so that baseline data could be collected during early pregnancy. It was hoped that these data would not be distorted by subsequent events or undermined so much by poor recollection.

METHOD

Data were collected in four waves. These are described briefly below and outlined in more detail later in this chapter.

WAVE ONE - 12 WEEKS PREGNANT

This phase of the study involved an interview using a standardized schedule, with 1,008 women. These respondents were interviewed at three antenatal clinics when approximately twelve weeks pregnant. A second instrument was employed to elicit additional data from clinic case notes. Blood tests, Gamma-Glutamyl-Transpeptidase (y-GT), and Mean Cell Volume (MCV) were carried out. It was hoped that these measures might help validate self-reported levels of alcohol consumption.

WAVE TWO - 34 WEEKS PREGNANT

The 1,008 women were divided into three sub-groups, high, medium and low, according to their self-reported levels of alcohol consumption at 12 weeks. Three hundred respondents were randomly selected to be re-interviewed at 34 weeks. Blood tests were again taken to help validate self-reported alcohol consumption. A second instrument elicited relevant details of the progress of pregnancy from clinic case notes.

WAVE THREE - PREGNANCY OUTCOME

By arrangement with the relevant clinics' medical staff, the researcher was provided with details of the precise outcomes of the 1,008 pregnancies. Information on pregnancies that did not result in live births was elicited from the mothers' case notes. The time of event, for example, spontaneous abortion, was noted.

WAVE FOUR - 12 WEEK CHECK OF SURVIVING BABIES

All respondents' surviving offspring were assessed for normal development when 3 months old. This was accomplished using reports from health visitors who carried out the appropriate examinations.

PRETESTING AND PILOTING

The phase one interview schedule was pretested upon six female members of staff at the Psychiatry Department of the University of Edinburgh, then with six of the researcher's friends who were pregnant or had recently had babies. No major problems being evident, the fieldwork procedure was piloted upon ten women attending one of the co-operating antenatal clinics. As noted above, this study involved four waves of data collection. A detailed account of the methods employed is now presented.

WAVE ONE – 12 WEEKS PREGNANT

The first phase of this study took place in one of Edinburgh's largest antenatal departments, the Simpson Memorial Maternity Pavilion. Three clinics within this institution were chosen for research because of the wide geographical area they covered. The women came from a wide variety of social classes, and were drawn from the Lothian Region, part of the South East of Scotland, and part of Fife. The co-operation of the nursing and medical staff was enlisted and interviews were obtained from 1,008 women who attended the three clinics consecutively, during the study period. The aims and methods of the study were explained to potential respondents who were then requested to participate. Full details of this phase of the study, including patterns of response, are provided in chapter 3.

Data were collected by standardized interview, by information obtained from clinic case notes and from blood tests. The standardized interview schedule (see Appendix I) was administered by one of five interviewers who had been specially trained for this purpose by the researcher. The interviewers were all women with children. These women were moderate drinkers. The respondents were made aware that the interviewers were not members of the clinic staff. They were identified as working with the Alcohol Research Group of Edinburgh University and they did not wear uniforms or white coats. The interview schedule was administered in a quiet place away from the main treatment area. The respondents were assured that the information collected would be treated confidentially, even though it was not anonymous, since the study involved follow-up procedures. The interview schedule included questions on the following topics.

(1) general biographical data: for example, birthplace, marital status, occupation
(2) drinking habits prior to and during pregnancy
(3) experience of alcohol-related problems
(4) experience of physical problems
(5) stress
(6) smoking habits
(7) other drug use, legal and illegal
(8) nutritional intake
(9) drinking habits and any drinking problems of parents and husband/boyfriend/cohabitee.

Full details of this interview schedule are provided in Appendix I.

The second instrument in the first wave was used to collect relevant material from clinic case notes. The information obtained included such items as:

(1) age
(2) height
(3) weight
(4) blood pressure
(5) urinalysis
(6) details of past obstetric history.

Each patient's case notes were clearly marked with a label that stated, 'This patient is taking part in the Alcohol Research Group study'. This aided later identification. Full details of this instrument are provided in Appendix I.

WAVE TWO – 34 WEEKS PREGNANT

As noted above, the respondents were divided into three sub-groups according to their levels of self-reported alcohol consumption. These sub-groups are defined in chapter 3. Data were obtained by employing similar procedures to those involved in wave one. A shortened version of the initial interview was administered. Additional data were elicited from clinic case notes. Some additional information was obtained for this second phase. This related to the patient's health in the current pregnancy, such as hospital admissions and reasons for these, together with details of any infections or other health problems, such as ankle oedema, with the prescribed treatment. Full details of this instrument are provided in Appendix II.

WAVE THREE - PREGNANCY OUTCOMES

This entailed a full examination of surviving offspring carried out by the paediatricians within 24 hours of birth. The information also included an account of the mother's pregnancy, with any problems, any drugs administered and, if so, when in the pregnancy. Also included was an account of the mother's labour, such as:

(1) onset of labour, for example, spontaneous or induced
(2) drugs given in labour
(3) mode of delivery, for example, vertex, breech
(4) any complications
(5) placental weight
(6) placental condition
(7) membrane rupture/delivery interval.

Information about the baby included:

(1) Apgar scores for 1 and 5 minutes
(2) any resuscitation necessary
(3) birth weight
(4) birth length
(5) occipito-frontal circumference
(6) full physical examination
(7) any abnormalities and their treatment
(8) any problems and their treatment
(9) type of feeding, for example breast or bottle.

The paediatricians knew the babies were part of the study as a label was attached to the babies' case notes, which read: 'This baby is taking part in the Alcohol Research Group study'. Even so, they did not have any information about the mothers' drinking. In this way, the examination of the babies was completed 'blind'. Data for this phase of the study were obtained from case notes by the project's clerical assistant, who completed a standardized instrument. Details of this are given in Appendix III. Data were also obtained on the outcomes of pregnancies that did not result in live births. Details of spontaneous abortions or terminations were recorded from the mothers' notes, along with the reasons and the week in pregnancy of this event. Stillbirths and neonatal deaths were recorded along with information from the postmortem reports.

WAVE FOUR - 12 WEEK CHECK OF SURVIVING BABIES

This phase of the study was carried out by the relevant health visitors. Prior to this, written consent to obtain this information had been sought and provided by the mothers' medical practitioners. Health visitors completed a brief standardized instrument (see Appendix IV). The instrument included information on the following.

(1)   weight
(2)   length
(3)   head circumference
(4)   palpebral fissure size
(5)   development check
(6)   feeding – breast or bottle
(7)   feeding problems, for example sucking difficulties
(8)   sleeping
(9)   general health.

The health visitors, like the paediatricians, were not informed of the drinking status of the mothers in this study.

THE SIZE OF THE STUDY GROUP

The size of the study group was chosen as sufficient to generate an adequate body of data related to alcohol consumption levels and to fetal alcohol *effects*. Some commentators (Hanson *et al.* 1978) have suggested that approximately one per 500 live births exhibits the features of the fetal alcohol syndrome. This estimate relates to 'normal populations'. It has been claimed that in more deprived settings, such as North American Indian reservations, the rate of the full-blown syndrome might be as high as one per seventy-two live births. This study was *not* designed to be a search for the full fetal alcohol syndrome. It was undertaken to look for fetal alcohol effects that in general populations are believed to be less serious and more commonplace at five or six per 1,000 live births.

CHOICE OF CLINICS

The three clinics were selected because the women attending them were drawn from the complete social spectrum. The clinics also appeared capable of yielding the required size of study group in an acceptable period of time. In fact, the initial wave of data collection took one year to complete and not six months as originally anticipated.

SELECTION OF INTERVIEWERS

It was decided that interviewers for the first two waves of the study would be specially recruited and trained for this purpose. In addition, these individuals were not to be clinic staff. This decision was taken after reference to available evidence about the type of interviewers who were most likely to obtain full information. Little states, 'These data suggest that the reports of drinking to the physician were of limited usefulness, because all women tended to declare similar quantities. Furthermore, physician interrogation failed to detect almost all the heavy drinkers found by an independent interviewer' (1976: 592).

SOME INITIAL DILEMMAS

Before the commencement of this study, three ethical and procedural issues were considered and resolved.
(1) What information, if any, was to be provided to respondents asking about the relationship between drinking during pregnancy and fetal harm?
(2) What advice, if any, was to be offered to respondents who did appear to be consuming 'dangerous' levels of alcohol?
(3) Were clinic staff to be granted access to data about respondents that were collected during this research project?
Respondents who did inquire about the general link between alcohol consumption during pregnancy and fetal harm were to be provided with the following brief factual statement. 'Evidence from America suggests that heavy drinking during pregnancy is harmful and the current study is being undertaken to ascertain at which levels of alcohol consumption damage might occur'.

The second dilemma was resolved only after a great deal of deliberation. It was decided that giving any advice to respondents about their drinking or related issues was inappropriate. Such advice might have biased the study. The issue of confidentiality required less heart searching to resolve. All of the information collected was confidential. In consequence, no details relating to individual respondents were made available to clinic staff. In fact, no such details were requested. Even so, it was decided that if clinic staff were concerned about an individual's drinking they could be advised upon how best to record histories of alcohol consumption. In addition, advice was made available to nursing and medical staff seeking information about local agencies providing help for problem drinkers.

THE VALIDITY OF ALCOHOL CONSUMPTION DATA

It has been widely noted that surveys of self-reported use and alcohol-related problems are afflicted by extensive under-reporting (Popham 1970: Pernanen 1974; Midanik 1982a). In relation to alcohol consumption, Pernanen has suggested that surveys only account for 40 to 60 per cent of known consumption. In addition, it has been suggested that under-reporting might be particularly great among those who are the heaviest drinkers (Schmidt 1972). Midanik (1982a) concluded that the validity of data from alcohol surveys varies in relation to the variables being recorded and to the methods adopted. Although most concern has related to under-reporting, Midanik (1982b) has noted that among a group of clinic problem drinkers, survey data were distorted by over-reporting. The question of validity is an issue of major importance in relation to alcohol consumption. Garrett and Barr (1974) found that men consistently underrated their drinking. In contrast, women generally perceived their drinking accurately or were just as likely to overestimate as underestimate their consumption. Cahalan and Treiman (1976) found no diferences between men and women when they were asked how likely they were to conceal their drinking. Barr *et al.* (1977) concluded that the inaccuracy and unreliability of reported consumption was more than three times as common among 16 to 17-year-old male high school students than among females of the same age.

Relevant evidence is limited and confused. None the less, it is reassuring for this study that females appear to be at least as accurate in their survey responses as are males. None the less, more general evidence about biases in such survey data is important and deserves recognition. Concern about self-reported data prompted the use of relevant blood tests in this study. It was hoped that these might provide an additional criterion by which alcohol consumption, especially heavy consumption, might be measured.

3 Baseline data

This chapter describes the findings from the first wave of the study.

RESPONSE OF THE STUDY GROUP

The total number of women interviewed was 1,008. In addition to these, thirty women agreed to take part in the project but, through lack of time on their part, combined with delay in completing the necessary antenatal procedures, they were unable to participate. A further ten women were excluded from the investigation because they could not speak English. Most of these were from the Indian subcontinent and were probably abstainers. Thirteen women refused to participate in the study. At least one of these had two damaged babies from previous pregnancies. The net response rate was therefore 95.0 per cent (1,008 out of 1,061). A minority of the study group were unable to answer some of the questions in the interview. In consequence, some of the totals presented below vary slightly.

BIOGRAPHICAL DATA

The majority of the women, 82.3 per cent, were between 21 and 35 years of age; 91.2 per cent were married, or cohabiting; a total of 80.1 per cent were Scots born; 53.0 per cent of the study group were working, and a further 42.8 per cent stated they were full-time housewives. A total of 51.8 per cent reported that their husbands, cohabitees, or boyfriends were manual workers. This corresponds closely with the general population of Edinburgh. The 1981 10 per cent sample Census showed that 50.0 per cent of married women in this city lived in households headed by a manual worker (Registrar General for Scotland 1984). Most of the study group, 55.7 per cent, had had at least one previous pregnancy.

SELF-REPORTED ALCOHOL CONSUMPTION

Eight per cent of the study group reported never having drunk alcohol.

RECENCY OF LAST DRINK

Respondents were asked when they had last consumed alcohol. The majority, 80.5 per cent, reported having drunk since becoming pregnant and 38.5 per cent had done so during the seven days preceding interview.

PREVIOUS WEEK'S CONSUMPTION

Those who had consumed alcohol in the previous week were asked to provide a detailed account of what they had drunk. This procedure has been widely used in earlier British studies. (Dight 1976: 588–92; Plant 1977: 54; Wilson 1980a: 1; Wilson 1980b: 14–16) The average consumption per drinker in the previous week was low, 3.5 units. However, twenty-two respondents, 5.7 per cent of those who had drunk in the previous week, reported drinking 10 or more units. One of these respondents reported that she had consumed 34 units. The majority, 67.8 per cent of those who had drunk in the previous week, reported having done so on one day only. A further 16.6 per cent had drunk on only two days. Eighty-three per cent of the study group reported that their previous week's alcohol consumption (or lack of it) was typical of what they had been drinking lately.

MAXIMUM DAILY ALCOHOL CONSUMPTION DURING PREGNANCY

Respondents were asked what was the maximum amount of alcohol they had consumed on any single day since becoming pregnant. Altogether, 789 respondents (78.3 per cent) provided details of this. The additional twenty-two women who reported having drunk during pregnancy failed to recall the quantities involved. The average level of consumption on this maximum drinking day during the first trimester of pregnancy was 4.4 units per drinker. The maximum amount reportedly consumed by any one respondent on this single day was 39 units. A total of 281 (35.6 per cent) of those providing details of their consumption reported having drunk 5 or more units. In addition, forty-seven women (6 per cent) of those providing details and 4.7 per cent of the entire study group reported having drunk 10 or more units. The patterns of self-reported alcohol consumption in the week preceding the interview and during the maximum drinking day in pregnancy are shown in *Figure 4*.

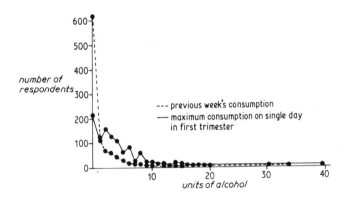

Figure 4 Patterns of alcohol consumption during week preceding interview and on maximum drinking day during first trimester of pregnancy

   The maximum day's consumption during the first trimester was significantly positively correlated both with the total consumption during the week preceding interview (r = +0.41; p < 0.001) and with maximum consumption on a single day during that week (r = +0.44; p < 0.001). (Pearson (Product-Moment) Correlation. All correlations are of this type unless stated otherwise.)

DRINKING BEFORE PREGNANCY

Respondents were asked how much they had consumed on a typical drinking day before pregnancy. The average amount reported by those who were drinkers was 3.7 units. The pattern of self-reported consumption before conception was significantly positively correlated both with previous week's consumption (r = +0.23; p < 0.001) and with the maximum day's level of consumption during the first trimester (r = +0.45; p < 0.001).

THE EFFECTS OF PREGNANCY ON DRINKING

Respondents were asked how their drinking since becoming pregnant compared with that before conception. The great majority (70.8 per cent) reported having reduced their consumption, while 27.9 per cent stated that their consumption was unaffected and 1.3 per cent stated that they were drinking more than before conception.

Strikingly, 52.3 per cent of those who reported having reduced their level of consumption since conception stated that they had done so out of concern that their previous level of drinking might harm their babies. Most of the remainder attributed their reduction to nausea (17.7 per cent) or to dislike of the taste of alcohol since conception (20.7 per cent). The main reasons identified for the increase were domestic problems or having been on holiday.

Two hundred and forty-eight women, 30.6 per cent of those who had drunk since conception, reported that they had noticed a change in the effect of alcohol upon them since pregnancy. The most common reported effect was nausea (N = 121). Fifty-seven respondents stated that alcohol affected them more quickly than formerly and forty-six stated that it tasted different.

INTOXICATION DURING PREGNANCY

One hundred and seventy-two respondents reported having at some time been 'merry, happy, or intoxicated' due to drinking since conception. These constituted 21.2 per cent of those who had consumed alcohol during the first trimester and 17.1 per cent of the entire study group.

The mean number of episodes of intoxication reported by these women was 1.7. Seventeen respondents reported having been merry, happy, or intoxicated four or more times since conception. These constituted 9.9 per cent of those who had consumed alcohol during the first trimester and 1.7 per cent of the entire study group.

CONSEQUENCES OF DRINKING

Data were obtained relating to fifteen questions concerning experience of some possible consequences of excessive drinking by the study group or by their close relatives. The reported levels of these consequences are shown in *Table 2*.

Table 2 Experience of alcohol-related consequences by the study group and their close relatives

Type of consequence (in rank order)	N	%
Father had experienced drinking problems	87	8.6
Have had gastritis	66	6.5
Have had 'liver trouble'	63	6.2
Husband has experienced drinking problems	29	2.9
Have been worried about own drinking	20	2.0
Have had peripheral neuritis	19	1.9
Mother had experienced drinking problems	19	1.9
Have had duodenal ulcer	12	1.2
Have had health problems due to drinking	6	0.6
Have had domestic problems due to drinking	5	0.5
Have had help for drinking problems	3	0.3
Have had legal problems due to drinking	2	0.2
Have had work problems due to drinking	2	0.2
Have had financial problems due to drinking	1	0.1

Percentages relate to the entire study group (N = 1,008)

As shown in *Table 2*, the direct or indirect consequences most commonly experienced were having a father who had experienced drinking problems (8.6 per cent) and having had gastritis (6.5 per cent).

Altogether, 277 (27.5 per cent) of the study group reported having experienced one or more of these consequences. Of these respondents, sixty-one (6 per cent) reported having experienced two of these consequences, three reported having experienced three of these consequences, four reported having experienced four consequences, and one had experience of six. Experience of these consequences was significantly (but slightly) positively correlated with previous week's alcohol consumption ($r = +0.08$; $p < 0.001$), maximum daily consumption during the previous week ($r = +0.12$; $p < 0.001$), maximum day's consumption during the first trimester ($r = +0.13$; $p < 0.001$).

SMOKING

Three hundred and forty-seven respondents, 34.4 per cent of the study group, reported that they currently smoked tobacco. An additional 145 women, 14.4 per cent, stated that they had smoked before conception, but had ceased to do so once they had discovered

64   *Women, Drinking, and Pregnancy*

that they were pregnant. Accordingly, only 29.5 per cent of the 492 women who smoked before pregnancy had stopped. Altogether, 228 women stated that they had smoked less than before they were pregnant. By far the commonest explanation for cessation or reduction in smoking, offered by 150 women, was fear that smoking might harm the fetus. Nausea was identified as the main explanation by a further thirty-three women. Smoking was not significantly correlated with frequency of maternal intoxication. However, smoking was significantly positively correlated with the number of alcohol-related consequences (r = +0.14; p < 0.001).

USE OF DRUGS

Two types of drugs were considered, apart from alcohol and tobacco. First, medicines, which included all prescribed and over-the-counter preparations. Second, illicit drugs. These were psychoactive substances, such as cannabis and heroin, which are controlled by the Misuse of Drugs Act (1971), as well as glues and solvents which, though legal, are generally regarded as drugs of misuse.

Thirteen respondents, 1.3 per cent of the study group, reported having used illicit drugs since conception. In marked contrast, 62.8 per cent of the study group reported having used some form of licit or prescribed drug during the first trimester. The extent of illicit and licit drug use is indicated in *Table 3*.

Table 3   Use of illicit drugs and licit or prescribed drugs during the first trimester by the study group

number of drugs used	illicit drugs		licit or prescribed drugs	
	N	%	N	%
0	995	98.7	375	37.2
1	12	1.2	403	40.0
2	1	0.1	174	17.3
3	–	–	45	4.5
4	–	–	11	1.1
total	1,008	100.0	1,008	100.0

The overwhelming majority of the study group reported having consumed some type of psychoactive substance since conception. This included alcohol, tobacco, illicit or licit and prescribed drugs.

Only 4.6 per cent of respondents stated that they had not ingested any of these substances during the first trimester.

CAFFEINE INTAKE

Almost half of the women in the study group, 44 per cent (439), reported consuming between one and four cups of coffee a day with a further 13 per cent (129) reportedly drinking between five and nine cups a day. Fifty-four per cent (544) of the group drank between one and four cups of tea daily with a further 22 per cent (225) consuming between five and nine cups.

STRESS

One hundred and sixty-eight (17 per cent) respondents reported having been under some kind of emotional stress since conception. The main reasons for stress were domestic problems (forty-nine respondents) and apprehension about the birth (twenty-nine respondents).

PARASUICIDE (ATTEMPTED SUICIDE)

Forty-two respondents, 4.2 per cent of the study group, reported that they had at some time taken an overdose. Five of these women had reportedly done so on more than one occasion.

BLOOD TESTS

As noted above, blood samples were taken from respondents from which MCV and y-GT values were obtained. The relationship between these tests and self-reported alcohol consumption was examined. Four possible confounding factors were controlled for. These were: the respondent's age; weight; smoking habits; and the occupational status of the respondent's spouse, boyfriend, or cohabitee.

Four measures of alcohol consumption were considered. These were: total previous week's consumption; maximum day's consumption during the previous week; maximum day's consumption during the first trimester, and typical drinking day's consumption before conception. MCV was significantly positively correlated with all four consumption measures. In contrast, y-GT was significantly positively correlated with only one: maximum day's consumption during the first trimester. The levels of correlations obtained are shown in *Table 4*.

Table 4   Correlations between blood tests and self-reported alcohol consumption

measure of self-reported alcohol consumption	type of blood test	
	MCV	y-GT
total previous week's consumption	+ 0.10**	NS
maximum day's consumption in previous week	+ 0.09**	NS
maximum day's consumption in first trimester	+ 0.07*	+ 0.08*
typical drinking day's consumption before conception	+ 0.10**	NS

* p < 0.05
** p < 0.01

PREVIOUS OBSTETRIC PROBLEMS

Details were obtained from clinic case notes of each respondent's obstetric history. This information related to previous stillbirths, spontaneous abortions, terminations, and to physically and mentally handicapped children already produced.

Two hundred and thirty-eight respondents, 23.6 per cent of the study group, were noted as having experienced one or more of these problems. Forty-six women had experienced two, eleven women had experienced three, and two women had experienced four problems. The overall levels of experience of these five types of problem are shown in *Table 5*.

Table 5   Experience of previous obstetric problems amongst the study group

type of problem	number experienced				total	
	1	2	3	4	N	%
stillbirths	10				10	1.0
spontaneous abortions	94	18	4	2	118	11.7
terminations	110	8	3		121	12.0
physically handicapped children	10	1			11	1.1
mentally handicapped children	5				5	0.5

As *Table 5* indicates, the obstetric problems that had been most commonly experienced were terminations (12 per cent) and spontaneous abortions (11.7 per cent).

THE ASSOCIATION BETWEEN PREVIOUS OBSTETRIC PROBLEMS AND
ALCOHOL CONSUMPTION

The relationship between each of the five types of previous problems and self-reported alcohol consumption was examined. This analysis was conducted by partial correlation, controlling for the possible confounding effects of respondent's age, smoking, illicit and licit drug use during the first trimester, and the occupational status of the respondent's husband, boyfriend, or cohabitee. The significant correlations between obstetric problems and alcohol consumption are presented in *Table 6*.

Table 6 Significant partial correlations between previous obstetric problems and self-reported alcohol consumption (all respondents)

measure of self-reported alcohol consumption	having had a stillbirth	having had a spontaneous abortion	having had a termination	having had a physically handicapped child	having had a mentally handicapped child
previous week's total consumption	+ 0.22***	+ 0.16***	+ 0.26***	+ 0.12***	+ 0.31***
maximum day's consumption in previous week	+ 0.13***	+ 0.08**	+ 0.21***	+ 0.14***	+ 0.20***
maximum day's consumption in first trimester	+ 0.06*	NS	+ 0.19***	+ 0.08**	+ 0.09**
typical day's consumption before pregnancy	− 0.05*	− 0.05*	NS	NS	− 0.05*

* p < 0.05
** p < 0.01
*** p < 0.001

A significant positive correlation emerged between having had a termination and having had a physically or mentally handicapped child, a stillbirth or a spontaneous abortion, and self-reported alcohol consumption. These were significantly positively correlated with previous week's consumption and maximum day's consumption during the previous week. In addition, all except having had a spontaneous abortion were also significantly correlated with maximum day's consumption during the first trimester.

In an attempt to establish whether factors other than alcohol were associated with fetal harm, the relationship between the intake of twelve types of food and non-alcoholic beverages to obstetric problems was examined. Three of these, coffee, liver, and milk, were significantly positively correlated with either spontaneous abortions, stillbirths, or terminations. Accordingly, an additional partial correlation was carried out to control for these possible confounding factors. The significant positive correlations between terminations, spontaneous abortions, stillbirth, physically or mentally handicapped children, noted in *Table 6*, survived almost unchanged.

The partial correlations depicted in *Table 6* were recalculated for 'drinkers' only. These were the 791 respondents who had consumed alcohol since conception. The results of this procedure are shown in *Table 7*.

Table 7 Significant correlations between previous obstetric problems and self-reported alcohol consumption (drinkers only)

measures of self-reported alcohol consumption	having had a stillbirth	having had a spontaneous abortion	having had a termination	having had a physically handicapped child	having had a mentally handicapped child
previous week's total consumption	NS	NS	+0.16***	+0.12***	+0.12***
maximum day's consumption in previous week	+0.13***	+0.09**	+0.23***	+0.14***	+0.22***
maximum day's consumption in first trimester	+0.04	NS	+0.20***	+0.14**	+0.07*
typical day's consumption before pregnancy	-0.07*	-0.07*	NS	NS	-0.07*

* p < 0.05
** p < 0.01
*** p < 0.001

As *Table 7* indicates, when abstainers were excluded, two of the original partial correlations ceased to be significant. These related to the associations between having had a stillbirth or spontaneous abortion and previous week's consumption. The remaining fifteen correlations remained significant, if small, with typical day's consumption before pregnancy again negatively correlated. The procedure illustrated by *Table 7* was repeated. This time, caffeine consumption was included in the variable 'licit and illicit drug use'. Nine of the fifteen significant correlations in *Table 7* remained significant.

The five separate measures of obstetric problems were combined. A further partial correlation was carried out to ascertain whether or not there was an association between the overall number of such problems and self-reported alcohol consumption. As before, the possible confounding factors of respondent's age, smoking, licit and illicit drug use, together with the occupational status of respondent's spouse, boyfriend, or cohabitee, were controlled for. This analysis, which related to the whole study group, revealed that there was a significant positive correlation between the overall level of obstetric problems experienced and maximum day's alcohol consumption in the week before interview ($r = +0.05$; $p < 0.05$). There was, however, no such significant correlation between the overall level of obstetric problems and total previous week's consumption, maximum day's consumption during the first trimester, or with typical drinking day's consumption before conception.

This procedure was repeated for drinkers only. Quite different results were produced. Significant positive correlations emerged between the overall level of obstetric problems and total previous week's drinking ($r = +0.06$; $p < 0.05$) and maximum day's consumption during the first trimester ($r = +0.07$; $p < 0.05$). This procedure was again repeated. Caffeine consumption was again included in the variable 'licit and illicit drug use'. This did not significantly alter the results noted above.

FAMILY HISTORY OF DRINKING PROBLEMS

Twenty-nine respondents (2.9 per cent) reported having husbands who had drinking problems. Fifteen of these were reportedly mainly health problems and fourteen were mainly domestic difficulties. The other family members about whom information was sought were parents. Eighty-seven respondents (8.6 per cent) reported having fathers who had drinking problems and nineteen respondents (1.9 per cent) reported having mothers who were problem drinkers.

COMPARISON WITH OTHER STUDIES

GENERAL LEVEL OF ALCOHOL CONSUMPTION

A survey has recently been conducted in Scotland that serves as a useful source of comparative data (Wilson 1980a). This study has already been briefly cited in the Introduction.

This related to a Scottish national random sample of 425 women who were interviewed during the autumn of 1978. This survey showed that the average previous week's self-reported alcohol consumption of women aged twenty and over, who had consumed alcohol during that period, was 6.2 units. This indicates that most respondents in the present study were not drinking heavily in relation to a more general population group. This view is consistent with the evidence cited above that 70.8 per cent of the study group reported having drunk less since conception than they had done before.

BLOOD TESTS

As *Table 4* indicates, the significant correlations noted between alcohol consumption and blood tests were low. The inter-correlations were markedly lower than those obtained by an earlier study in the same locality (Chick *et al.* 1981). These had produced correlations of + 0.42 and + 0.36 respectively, between y-GT and MCV and previous week's alcohol consumption. The earlier study related to males who were much heavier drinkers than the present study group. Even so, Chick *et al.* had noted that: 'for screening, however, these tests appear to lack power' (1981: 1251). A study of pregnant women in London (Barrison *et al.* 1982) states: 'These findings show that mean cell volume is not a valuable measure of potentially harmful drinking during pregnancy and that y-glutamyl transpeptidase is only of limited value in the first trimester' (1982: 1318). This conclusion appears to be corroborated even more forcefully by the present results. It is concluded that the tests have little value in relation to the study group's generally modest levels of alcohol consumption.

DRUG USE

Studies on drug use in pregnancy show the percentage of women taking prescribed, over-the-counter, and illicit drugs varies greatly. As Rayburn states: 'A drug-free pregnancy is ideal but drug surveys indicate that despite "therapeutic restraints" 90 per cent or more of all pregnant women take one or more drugs during pregnancy in addition to dietary supplements' (Rayburn *et al.* 1982: 569). The baseline results of the present study are consistent with this conclusion.

CAFFEINE CONSUMPTION

The levels of coffee consumption noted in this study were higher than those described by Hartwig *et al.* (1982) in Berlin. Sixty-six per cent of their respondents were consuming one or two cups of coffee daily. However, the results of the present study are similar to those obtained by Kuzma (1982) who reported that 48 per cent of his study group consumed between one and six cups of coffee daily. The relationship between caffeine consumption and fetal harm is still questionable. In fact, according to Linn *et al.* (1982) in their study of 12,205 women, an analysis of coffee consumption and outcome of pregnancy did not reveal any relationship between prematurity or incidence of malformation and coffee consumption after they controlled for tobacco use. The relationship between caffeine consumption and fetal harm needs to be examined more closely. However, this was not an aim of this study and is only noted again briefly in chapters 5 and 6.

OBSTETRIC PROBLEMS

As noted in chapter 1, previous studies, while sometimes indicating that consumption is associated with increased risks of harm, are by no means uniform in their conclusions about the levels and patterns of alcohol consumption at which this occurs. Four of the studies cited in chapter 1 are particularly relevant to the present investigation since they collected alcohol consumption data during pregnancy (Kuzma 1976; Kaminsky *et al.* 1976; Little 1977; Harlap and Shiona 1980; Streissguth *et al.* 1981; and Rosett *et al.* 1976). These investigations all obtained their alcohol consumption data by some form of quantity-frequency index, and not, as in the present study, primarily from an analysis of previous week's drinking. As noted by Duffy (1982) there are major differences between these two approaches and in some respects the latter is the more precise. Even so, it is of interest to make some comparisons between the earlier investigations and the present study.

The lowest level of daily drinking reported to be harmful (Harlap and Shiona) was 1.5 units. This is equivalent to a weekly total of 10.5 units, which has reportedly been exceeded by 18 respondents, 1.8 per cent in the present study group. Kline *et al.* (1980) reported that there was a serious risk of spontaneous abortion among mothers who consumed the equivalent of 3 units of alcohol on at least two occasions per week. As indicated by *Figure 4*, 8 per cent of the study group had exceeded this level on at least one day during the week preceding interview. Streissguth *et al.* (1981) reported that binge drinking was associated with decreased birth weight. The definition of a binge was 'a day (or more) when drinking was at least double the regular level and a minimum of 3 oz of absolute alcohol was consumed'.

As indicated by *Figure 4*, forty-eight respondents, 4.8 per cent of the study group, reported having consumed 10 units or more on a single day during the first trimester, which could reasonably be defined as a binge. Fifteen of these women, 1.5 per cent of the study group, reported that their maximum day's consumption during pregnancy had been 15 units or more. As noted in chapter 1, other studies have reported that an association is evident between even lower levels of alcohol consumption and fetal harm than those noted in the four studies above.

SUMMARY

This chapter reports only retrospective baseline results. The primary focus of this study relates to the prospective data that are described in the following three chapters. Chapters 5 and 6, which are related to pregnancy outcomes and to the follow-up of babies, are crucial to the aims of this investigation. These initial baseline findings indicate that the self-reported alcohol consumption of the study group was significantly positively correlated with previous obstetric problems. However, considering the size of the study group, these correlations, though significant, are extremely weak. Previous obstetric problems, though associated with alcohol consumption, may not be caused or even influenced by it. Even so, it is possible that women who are heavy drinkers are slightly more at risk of encountering obstetric difficulties.

4 Changes in alcohol consumption during pregnancy

As noted in chapter 2, the second wave of data collection involved re-interviewing a sub-sample of women during the thirty-fourth week of pregnancy. This phase of the study took place between July 1980 and November 1981. The main aim of this procedure was to ascertain whether or not levels of self-reported alcohol consumption change later in pregnancy.

METHOD

Two instruments were used in this wave of fieldwork. These were shortened versions of those employed in the initial data collection. The first was a short standardized interview. This was administered by one of two fieldworkers. The interview schedule included information on respondents' alcohol consumption, smoking, stress, use of medicines and illicit drugs, consumption of tea and coffee, and dietary intake. (See Appendix II(a) for full details.) The second method involved eliciting information from the respondents' clinical case notes. As during the first phase of the study, this procedure was conducted by trained fieldworkers. The document completed included information on problems in pregnancy, weight, and blood pressure (see Appendix II(b) for full details).

A sub-sample of 300 respondents was selected by the following procedure: using the approach adopted in the previous chapter the complete study group was divided into three sub-groups. This was done on the basis of their maximum day's alcohol consumption since conception. These sub-groups were: abstainers: those who had consumed no alcohol since conception (n = 219: 21.7 per cent); light drinkers: those who had consumed between one and four units on maximum drinking day since conception (n = 509: 50.3 per cent); heavy drinkers: those who had consumed five or more units on this occasion (n = 282: 28.0 per cent).

In order to give due weight to all of these sub-groups, respondents were arranged within each by their fieldwork code numbers. A systematic random selection of every third individual within each sub-group was made until the following numbers had been obtained: 65 abstainers, 151 light drinkers and 84 heavy drinkers. These numbers represent the appropriate proportions of each sub-group within the total study group.

RESULTS

Data were obtained from 255 respondents. The distribution of these within the three sub-groups is shown in *Table 8*.

Table 8   Patterns of response during the second wave of data collection

sub-group	respondents interviewed	non contacts
	N	N
abstainers	51	14
light drinkers	128	23
heavy drinkers	76	8
total	255 (85.0%)	45 (15%)

As shown by *Table 8* the net response rate was 85.0 per cent. Altogether, sixteen respondents had delivered early, eight respondents had left the study area and could not be re-interviewed at the appropriate time, and four had spontaneously aborted. In addition, twelve respondents refused to be interviewed on the grounds of having insufficient time to spare during their visit to the clinic.

The three sub-groups were chosen by assessment of maximum alcohol consumption since conception, but this procedure also produced a sub-sample that was representative of previous week's alcohol consumption. Two measures of the alcohol consumption data obtained at 12 weeks were compared with the same two alcohol consumption measures at 22 weeks. The results of this comparison are shown in *Table 9*.

Table 9 Changes in average levels of self-reported alcohol consumption in pregnancy

alcohol consumption measures	at 12 weeks pregnant	at 34 weeks pregnant	product-moment correlation between 12 weeks and 34 weeks
previous week's consumption*	1.5	1.1	r = + 0.63***
maximum day's consumption in the previous week*	1.0	0.7	r = + 0.53***

* Consumption is measured in units of alcohol.
*** p < 0.001

As indicated by *Table 9*, the average previous week's consumption had decreased slightly between the two points, from 1.5 units to 1.1 units. The maximum day's consumption in the previous week had also decreased from 1.0 to 0.7 units. Even so, both measures were quite highly intercorrelated. The patterns of alcohol consumption in the week preceding the interview and during the maximum day in the past 22 weeks are shown in *Figure 5*.

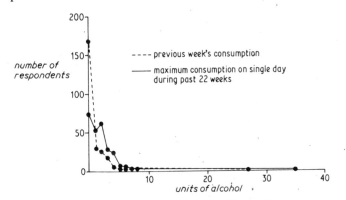

Figure 5 Patterns of alcohol consumption during week preceding second interview and on maximum drinking day during past 22 weeks of pregnancy

As indicated by *Figure 5*, the majority of respondents in this sub-sample, 165 (65 per cent), had consumed no alcohol in the previous week, the two heaviest drinkers had consumed 22 units and 27 units in that period. In terms of maximum day's consumption in the past 22 weeks, 72 respondents (28 per cent) consumed no alcohol, the majority, 113 respondents (44 per cent) of this sub-sample consumed between 1 and 2 units. The heaviest drinker consumed 35 units.

The general changes in previous week's alcohol consumption between waves one and two were as follows. Altogether, 18.4 per cent of the sub-group were drinking more; 25.5 per cent were drinking less; and 56.1 per cent reported that their consumption, or lack of it, remained unchanged.

Table 10 Significant correlations between variables at 34 weeks and measures of self-reported alcohol consumption and intoxication

variables	total previous week's consumption	maximum day's consumption in previous week	maximum day's consumption in last 22 weeks	frequency of intoxication
time of last drink	− 0.35***	− 0.48***	− 0.11*	− 0.29***
number of drinking days in previous week	+ 0.65***	+ 0.56***	+ 0.13*	+ 0.35***
total previous week's consumption		+ 0.80***	+ 0.56***	+ 0.69***
maximum day's consumption in the previous week	+ 0.80***		+ 0.69***	+ 0.41***
number of drinking days in the previous week	+ 0.62***	+ 0.53***	+ 0.39***	+ 0.30***
frequency of intoxication	+ 0.56***	+ 0.41***	+ 0.68***	
maximum day's consumption in previous 22 weeks	+ 0.74***	+ 0.69***		+ 0.68***
number of cigarettes smoked	+ 0.15*	+ 0.14*	+ 0.19**	+ 0.15**
stress due to domestic problems	NS	− 0.11*	NS	NS
stress caused by previous spontaneous abortion or stillbirth	+ 0.33***	NS	NS	NS
use of antacids	NS	NS	− 0.11*	NS
coffee consumption	+ 0.16*	+ 0.19**	NS	NS
number of hospital admissions	NS	− 0.11*	NS	NS
previous week's consumption in first 12 weeks of pregnancy	+ 0.63***	+ 0.55***	+ 0.50***	+ 0.31***
maximum day's consumption in first 12 weeks of pregnancy	+ 0.29***	+ 0.32***	+ 0.40***	+ 0.32***
typical day's drinking before pregnancy	+ 0.34***	+ 0.34***	+ 0.45***	+ 0.38***

* p < 0.05
** p < 0.01
*** p < 0.001

The relationship was examined between the variables in this wave of data collection and four alcohol-consumption measures. These were total previous week's consumption, maximum day's consumption in the previous week, maximum day's consumption in the past 22 weeks and frequency of intoxication in the past 22 weeks.

Forty of the ninety-two variables examined were significantly correlated with at least one measure of alcohol consumption. *Table 10* presents details of the sixteen variables that were so correlated at the level of r = 0.1 or above.

As shown by *Table 10* the main measures of self-reported alcohol consumption at 34 weeks were quite highly intercorrelated and were also fairly highly positively correlated with 'baseline' alcohol consumption measures obtained during the first phase of this study.

INTOXICATION DURING PREGNANCY

Five respondents, 0.5 per cent, reported having been merry, happy, or intoxicated once or twice in the past 22 weeks. Consistent with the results noted in chapter 3, the frequency of intoxication was significantly positively correlated with total previous week's consumption (r = +0.56; p < 0.001) and maximum day's consumption in the previous week (r = +0.41, p < 0.001).

SMOKING

Seventy-seven respondents, 30 per cent of the sub-sample, reported that they currently smoked tobacco. Eleven of these women, 4 per cent of this sub-sample, remarkably, reported having *started* smoking within the second trimester of pregnancy.

USE OF DRUGS

Following the approach described in the previous chapter, use of two broad categories of drugs was examined. These were medicines and illicit drugs. The former included all prescribed and over-the-counter preparations ranging from antibiotics to simple headache pills. The latter category were 'illicit drugs', these included all illegal substances such as cannabis and the opiates as well as glues and solvents.

The most commonly used types of medicines were antacids. These had been used by 133 respondents, 44 per cent of this sub-sample. In addition, 77 respondents, 30 per cent of the sub-sample, had used analgesics, and 40 respondents, 16 per cent of the sub-sample, had been prescribed antibiotics. Only three respondents reported illicit drug use during pregnancy. Two of these reported using cannabis, and one reported using morphine.

CAFFEINE INTAKE

Almost half of the sub-sample, 49 per cent (126), reported drinking between one and four cups of coffee a day. A further thirty-two respondents (13 per cent) reported consuming between five and nine cups a day. More than half of the respondents, 58 per cent (147), reported consuming one to four cups of tea, 21 per cent (53) reported consuming five to nine cups.

STRESS

Thirty-seven (15 per cent) respondents reported experiencing some kind of emotional stress within the previous 22 weeks. The main reasons given for such stress, as noted in the previous chapter, were domestic problems (fourteen respondents) and apprehension about the approaching birth (six respondents).

COMPARISON WITH OTHER STUDIES

In a study of 183 women, conducted by Little *et al.* (1976) in America, the subjects were interviewed in the fourth month of pregnancy. One hundred and fifty-six of these women were re-interviewed four months later. This revealed that 36 per cent of the women were drinking more, compared with only 18 per cent of those in the present study. Forty per cent were drinking less than during early pregnancy, this compares with only 25 per cent of these in the present study group. The majority (70 per cent) were drinking daily.

   Clearly, the respondents in the present study were drinking much less than those in Little's study, since most of the present study group did not drink daily.

SUMMARY

This chapter briefly describes the second wave of this study. The principal focus of this phase was the way in which alcohol consumption changed during pregnancy. It emerged that the general level of self-reported alcohol consumption of the sub-sample declined during pregnancy.

The effects of heavy drinking in pregnancy have been assessed by Rosett *et al.* in their Boston study. They stated:

'Among a group of 69 pregnant women who drank heavily, 25 reduced alcohol consumption before the third trimester. Infants born to these women showed less growth retardation than did infants born to 44 women who continued to drink heavily throughout the pregnancy. Analysis of other risk factors showed little effect on outcome when third trimester drinking patterns were held constant.'

(Rosett *et al.* 1980: 178)

The average level of alcohol consumption noted in the present study could not be compared with Rosett's sample of heavy drinkers who were drinking five or six drinks on some occasions and at least forty-five drinks per month. However, in Rosett's small sample of women who reduced their drinking, it does appear that their reduction in *heavy* drinking during the third trimester meant that fewer of these respondents' offspring had weight, length, or head circumference below the 10th percentile. For moderate drinking women, the efficacy of reduction of consumption during the latter part of pregnancy is as yet unproven.

5 *Pregnancy outcome*

The third wave of data collection was related to assessing the outcome of the 1,008 pregnancies in this study. This was carried out between May 1981 and July 1982. A total of 929 (92.9 per cent) of the pregnancies resulted in live births, and eight (0.8 per cent) in stillbirths. The results of the remaining 75 respondents' pregnancies were as follows: 39 respondents (3.9 per cent) were not traced, and 32 respondents (3.2 per cent) experienced spontaneous abortions. In addition, three respondents (0.9 per cent) did not return to the clinic and one had a termination of pregnancy due to a serious fetal abnormality. These outcomes are summarized in *Table 11*.

Table 11 Outcome of pregnancy

outcome of pregnancy	number*	pregnancies of the study group
		%
live birth	929	91.8
spontaneous abortion	32	3.2
termination for fetal abnormalities	1	0.1
stillbirths	8	0.8
mother cancelled appointment at clinic – no further information	3	0.3
moved/no trace	39	3.9
total	1012*	100.1

*Note: four sets of twins were produced.

Four of the respondents produced twins. To facilitate the comparison of mothers and babies, the information about these four women was duplicated. The size of the study group was increased accordingly from 1,008 to 1,012 (as indicated by *Table 11*). Data were collected from the babies' case records by two interviewers. The schedule employed during this wave of the study included information on the mother's pregnancy, labour record and drugs administered during labour, the mode of delivery, length of time between membrane rupture and delivery, and the placental weight and condition. The information on the baby included weight, length and head circumference, a full physical examination, Apgar scores for 1 and 5 minutes, resuscitation, evidence of jaundice, infections and general condition (see Appendix III for full details).

The measurement of palpebral fissure length, allegedly a feature of the fetal alcohol syndrome, was added to this extensive examination that was routinely carried out by the paediatricians within 24 hours of the baby's birth. Unfortunately, due to the change-over in medical staff and the already prolonged conventional examination, this addition was frequently missed. Accordingly, two research assistants were employed to measure the palpebral fissure length. They followed up the first eighty-five babies from whom this had been omitted and recorded this measurement. After this, the health visitors who carried out the fourth and final wave of data collection routinely measured the palpebral fissure lengths of the remaining babies in the study group.

RESULTS

The data collected during wave three were initially related to the self-reported alcohol consumption of the study group recorded during the first wave of the investigation. Of the ninety-six variables thus investigated, only ten were significantly associated with at least one of the four measures of alcohol consumption. The numbers of these abnormalities exhibited by the surviving offspring of the study group are shown in *Table 12*.

A total of 23.9 per cent of the surviving offspring in the study group had one alcohol-related abnormality, 15.3 per cent had two or more. It is emphasized that many of these features, such as mild jaundice or low birth weight, were trivial.

Table 12 The number of alcohol-related abnormalities in surviving offspring

number of abnormalities

	N	%
0	563	60.8
1	221	23.9
2	105	11.3
3	19	2.1
4	13	1.4
5	3	0.3
6	2	0.2
total	926	100.0

The relationship was examined between maternal alcohol consumption and both birth abnormalities and perinatal problems. The results are shown in *Tables 13, 14,* and *15*. Partial correlations were computed for each continuous third wave variable in relation to 4 measures of alcohol consumption. These related to total consumption in the previous week, maximum day's consumption in the previous week, maximum day's consumption in the first twelve weeks of pregnancy, and typical day's drinking before pregnancy. This procedure simultaneously controlled for age, smoking habits, consumption of medicines and illicit drugs, and the occupational status of each respondent's husband, boyfriend, or cohabitee. The results of this are shown in *Tables 13* and *14*. Ten perinatal problems were dichotomous. The relationship of these to baseline alcohol consumption was examined using two-tailed T-tests. The results of this procedure are shown in *Table 15*.

The levels of association between these abnormalities and self-reported maternal alcohol consumption are shown in *Tables 13, 14,* and *15*. *Table 13* relates to six birth abnormalities and *Tables 14* and *15* relate to four perinatal difficulties.

As shown, in *Tables 13, 14,* and *15*, eight of the ten variables were significantly associated with total consumption in the previous week, and six were significantly associated with maximum day's consumption in the first trimester. Two were significantly associated with typical day's consumption before pregnancy, and seven were associated with maximum day's alcohol consumption in the previous week.

Most of the 'significance' indicated by *Tables 13, 14,* and *15* was due to the alcohol consumption of mothers whose offspring had doubtful or borderline rather than definite abnormalities. The next

Table 13 Birth abnormalities which correlated significantly with baseline alcohol consumption measures

variable	total previous week's consumption	maximum consumption in one day in previous week	maximum consumption in one day in first trimester of pregnancy	typical day's consumption before pregnancy
baby's head	NS	NS	NS	+ .06*
baby's eyes	+ 0.23***	+ 0.12***	NS	NS
baby's mouth sounds	+ 0.18***	+ 0.11***	+ 0.1***	NS
baby's chest ausculation	+ 0.18***	NS	NS	NS
baby's spleen	+ 0.20***	+ 0.16***	+ 0.07*	NS
birthweight	– 0.13***	– 0.14***	– 0.11***	NS

* $p < 0.05$
** $p < 0.01$
*** $p < 0.001$

Table 14 Perinatal problems which correlated significantly with baseline alcohol consumption measures (continuous variables)

variable	total previous week's consumption	maximum day's consumption in previous week	maximum day's consumption in first trimester of pregnancy	typical day's consumption before pregnancy
jaundice	+ 0.41***	+ 0.29***	+ 0.17***	NS
Agpar score at 1 minute	– 0.18***	– 0.10***	– 0.07*	NS
Agpar score at 5 minutes	– 0.44***	– 0.30***	– 0.17***	NS

* $p < 0.05$
** $p < 0.01$
*** $p < 0.001$

Table 15 Perinatal problem which was significantly associated with baseline alcohol consumption: T-test (Dichotomous variable)

variable		Typical day's consumption before pregnancy		
Infection		Without problems	With problems	T Value
	$\overline{X}$	3.4 units	5.2 units	
	SD	2.5 units	2.6 units	2.89**
	N	897	16	

** $p < 0.01$; degrees of freedom = 911 (pooled variance).
Note: When alcohol consumption data were log-converted, this was still significant ($p < 0.01$).

stage of the analysis employed a more vigorous approach to these
data by examining the relationships of maternal drinking and other
factors to definite abnormalities. This revealed a much smaller link
between alcohol and pregnancy outcomes.

Combining the ten items included in *Tables 13, 14,* and *15,* a full
babies' problem scale was compiled. The relationship of this scale to
self-reported maternal alcohol consumption was then examined.
Partial correlations were calculated, controlling simultaneously for
respondent's age, smoking, legal and illicit drug use, together with
the occupational status of respondent's husband, boyfriend, or
cohabitee. This revealed that the scale of birth abnormalities was
only weakly associated with a typical day's alcohol consumption
before pregnancy.

It is emphasized that this scale related only to definite abnormalities. Each individual abnormality was given a value of one so that a
child with three abnormalities had a score of three.

The prevalence of the ten birth abnormalities contained in
Tables 13, 14, and *15* was examined in relation to three sub-groups
of respondents. These were abstainers, light drinkers, and heavy
drinkers. As in chapter 4, these sub-groups were defined in relation
to the maximum drinking day since conception. Abstainers had
consumed no alcohol since becoming pregnant. Light drinkers had
consumed between 1 and 4 units and heavy drinkers had consumed
5 or more on their maximum drinking day in this period.

As noted above, 39.9 per cent of the surviving babies were noted
to have one or more abnormal features. A dichotomy was made
between those who had either no abnormalities or one such feature,
and those who exhibited two or more.

Table 16 Risk of birth abnormalities by drinking status of mother

drinking status of mother	babies with two or more abnormalities	
	N	% of each sub-group
abstainers (n = 200)	22	11.0
light drinkers (n = 463)	73	15.8
heavy drinkers (n = 263)	47	17.9

(x^2 = 4.26; df = 2; NS)

As *Table 16* shows, the proportion of babies with two or more
abnormalities was not significantly higher among the heavy
drinkers than among other respondents.

Even so, the risk of producing a baby with two or more abnormal features was 62.7 per cent higher among heavy drinkers than among abstainers, and 13.3 per cent higher among heavy than among light drinkers. This conclusion is particularly striking since the definition of 'heavy drinker' was related to only 5 or more units in the week preceding interview. This is a modest quantity of alcohol.

In order to explore the upper end of the alcohol consumption range, the analysis in *Table 16* was repeated. This analysis examination used a more rigorous definition of 'heavy drinker' as one whose maximum day's alcohol consumption during the first trimester was 10 or more units. This did produce a significant result.

Table 17 Risk of birth abnormalities by maximum day's alcohol consumption during the first trimester

maximum day's consumption during the first trimester	babies with two or more abnormalities	
	N	% of each sub-group
no alcohol consumed (n = 200)	22	11.0
1–9 units consumed (n = 681)	104	15.3
10 units or more consumed (n = 45)	16	35.6

$(x^2 = 17.07: df = 2; p < 0.001)$

Referring to *Table 17*, those respondents whose day's consumption during the first trimester had been 10 or more units had a much increased risk of producing babies with two or more abnormalities. This risk was three times that of the abstainers and twice over that of those whose maximum day's consumption had been between 1 and 9 units.

Thus, maximum day's alcohol consumption since conception was significantly associated with the birth of a baby with two or more abnormalities. Birth damage was not significantly associated with previous week's alcohol consumption.

The study group were overwhelmingly 'light drinkers'. A substantial proportion of them, 39.1 per cent, had borne offspring with one or more of the ten 'alcohol-related abnormalities'. It is perhaps not surprising that the general level of such abnormalities (often trivial) and alcohol consumption in the previous week (generally low) were not significantly related when examined by partial correlation. In addition, as noted in chapter 1, it is possible that alcohol-related harm would be more attributable to maximum levels of alcohol consumption early in pregnancy rather than to that evident in the week preceding interview at 12 weeks pregnant, by which time the woman would be aware of her pregnancy. The significant differences shown in *Table 17* are informative since they relate to a sub-group of respondents whose drinking was extremely unusual. The analysis so far shows that some birth abnormalities were individually slightly associated with maternal alcohol consumption. The overall number of abnormalities, however, was not significantly associated with self-reported maternal alcohol consumption, either during or before the first 3 months of pregnancy. In addition, as shown by *Table 16*, mothers who were 'heavy' drinkers were not significantly more likely to have offspring with two or more abnormalities than were light drinkers or abstainers. In spite of this, heavy drinkers did have an increased risk of such abnormalities when compared to other respondents. This conclusion is supported by the data in both *Tables 16* and *17*. In addition, as shown in *Table 17*, respondents with higher peak levels of alcohol consumption (maximum day) during the first trimester had a significantly higher proportion of babies with two or more abnormalities. These results are broadly compatible with those of some of the studies reviewed in chapter 1.

Alcohol consumption is only one of the countless possible influences upon pregnancy outcome. Such associations do not by themselves provide any clue to the possible role of alcohol consumption as an influence upon this outcome. Clarifying the relative importance of alcohol in this respect was the key reason for conducting this investigation.

In order to evaluate the relationship of the 'alcohol-related' abnormalities scale to some of the 'key' variables collected during the first wave of data, an analysis was implemented by stepwise multiple regression. Thirty-one variables were included. The results of this procedure are shown in *Table 18*.

These variables combined to give only a very poor prediction in relation to birth abnormalities. Together, the variables only accounted for 6.1 per cent of the variance. The items that were most highly correlated with abnormalities, and that explained the greatest variance, were history of live births and previous terminations. Maternal height added 0.8 per cent and smoking explained 0.4 per cent. The only alcohol consumption measures that contributed to the variance were maximum day's consumption in the previous week and in the first trimester. These added less than 1.0 per cent.

Table 18 Stepwise multiple regression of predictors of birth abnormalities

independent variables	multiple correlations	variance accounted for
		%
previous livebirths	0.15	2.2
previous terminations of pregnancy	0.19	3.8
maternal height	0.21	4.4
smoking	0.22	4.8
diet: milk consumption	0.22	5.0
diet: tea consumption	0.23	5.2
use of medicines/legal drugs	0.23	5.3
number of previous pregnancies	0.23	5.4
illicit drug use	0.23	5.5
maternal age	0.24	5.6
diet: meat consumption	0.24	5.6
diet: fruit consumption	0.24	5.7
abnormal urine test	0.24	5.7
marital status	0.24	5.8
maximum day's alcohol consumption in previous week	0.24	5.8
maximum day's alcohol consumption since conception	0.24	5.9
social class	0.24	5.9
previous overdoses	0.24	5.9
high maternal blood pressure	0.24	6.0

Note: In view of the skewed distribution of abnormalities, the scale was square root converted for this analysis.

Other variables included milk consumption and all legal and illicit drug use. This analysis was repeated with only fifteen independent variables. These explained only 4.8 per cent of the variance, of which alcohol explained less than 1.0 per cent. This 'shortened' regression was repeated again but in relation solely to the offspring of women whose maximum day's alcohol consumption since conception had exceeded nine units. This explained 26.2 per cent of the variance. Social class explained 7.7 per cent and illegal drug use explained 7.1 per cent. Alcohol was again unimportant.

This analysis is of crucial significance to the interpretation of the results of this study. Some birth abnormalities were slightly associated with maternal alcohol consumption as shown by *Tables 13, 14, 15,* and *17.* Nevertheless, it appears from the results of these multiple regressions that these associations were not explained, except to a trivial degree, by either maternal alcohol consumption or by use of legal drugs. The use of tobacco and illegal drugs came out as greater predictors than any of these variables.

One of the aims of this study was to ascertain whether or not birth abnormalities constituted a syndrome. In order to investigate this, a factor analysis was conducted. This involved forty-nine variables. These included twenty-two types of birth abnormalities, fourteen difficulties in the perinatal period, and thirteen variables related to the mother. Those relating to birth abnormalities and perinatal difficulties had each been noted in three or more of the babies in the study. Variables relating to fewer infants were excluded. The thirteen variables relating to the mother included baseline data, such as maximum alcohol consumption in one day in the previous week, maximum day's consumption in the first trimester, typical drinking day's consumption before pregnancy, smoking, and other drug use.

The analysis was conducted to ascertain if any particular grouping of the variables had enough in common to constitute specific factors. A factor can be loosely defined as the outcome of discovering a group of variables having a certain characteristic. Sixteen factors emerged. However, no clear-cut constellation of alcohol consumption and fetal harm variables was evident (for full details see Appendix V). There was no indication that specific birth abnormalities clustered with maternal alcohol consumption data. Similar results were obtained when a second factor analysis was conducted in which only the ten alcohol-related abnormalities and 'baseline' items relating to the mothers were included.

COMPARISON WITH OTHER STUDIES

In order to compare this study with earlier work in the field a stepwise multiple regression was carried out in which birth weight was the dependent variable. This particular item was chosen because Kuzma and Sokol (1982) had used it for the same analysis. In order to facilitate comparison, eight independent variables were selected. The results of this exercise are shown in *Table 19*.

This comparison indicates that the present study and that by Kuzma provided broadly compatible results. In both studies duration of gestation was, not surprisingly, by far the most highly predictive of the independent variables. This explained 19.8 per cent of the variance in Kuzma's study, and 20.4 per cent of that in the present investigation. A perfect comparison of alcohol use in the two studies was not possible. Kuzma recorded details of the frequency with which three separate types of beverage alcohol had been consumed.

Table 19 Stepwise multiple regression of birthweight

Kuzma and Sokol 1982		Plant 1985	
independent variables	variance explained	independent variables	variance explained
	%		%
duration of gestation	19.8	duration of gestation	20.4
cigarette use	21.9	cigarette use	24.6
caffeine use	22.1	maximum day's alcohol	25.1
frequency of wine use	22.1	consumption in first	
frequency of liquor use	22.1	trimester	
parity	22.6	parity	25.6
previous spontaneous	22.8	maximum day's alcohol	25.9
abortions			
frequency of beer use	22.9	consumption in	
frequency of illicit	22.9	previous week	
drug use		previous spontaneous	26.1
		abortions	
		medicine use	26.2
		caffeine use	26.4
		illicit drug use	26.4

Nevertheless, in the present study, maximum day's alcohol consumption during the first trimester explained 0.5 per cent of the variance, and Kuzma's three alcohol variables explained 0.1 per cent. Cigarette use explained 4.2 per cent of the variance in the present study and 2.1 per cent of that in Kuzma's investigation. 'Substance use' (including alcohol) accounted for 5.3 per cent of the variance in the present study and 2.4 per cent of that in Kuzma's investigation.

Rosett *et al.* (1983) also used a similar analysis in which birth weight was the dependent variable. Their results showed '33 per cent of the variance was explained by gestational age. Prepregnancy weight, heavy drinking, baby's sex, race, cigarette smoking, education and parity . . . contributed 11 per cent to the variance' (Rosett *et al.* 1983: 542).

SUMMARY

Several maternal labour problems, birth abnormalities, and perinatal difficulties were individually significantly associated with self-reported alcohol consumption. Some earlier studies related to this subject have controlled for such variables as age, occupational status, smoking habits, and use of drugs other than alcohol. Some have confined their analysis to noting associations between alcohol consumption and pregnancy outcome, while controlling for such factors. Like the present study, these have indicated that maternal drinking is indeed *associated* with some individual birth abnormalities and other undesirable measures of pregnancy outcome. Further exploration of the data collected by the present study was conducted in an attempt to clarify the predictive power of the baseline data in relation to pregnancy outcomes.

Streissguth *et al.* also used multiple regression analysis in their Seattle study. The researchers state: 'Despite the significant alcohol effects it should be pointed out that the multiple correlations ranged from 0.27 to 0.34; thus, the variables considered in these regressions account for only about 5 per cent of the total variance between babies' (1980: 156). These findings show alcohol explaining slightly more of the variance than in this present study. Nevertheless, neither this present study nor the Seattle investigation appear to show clearly that alcohol is strongly predictive of fetal harm.

As noted above, in the present study, analysis revealed that although alcohol consumption was slightly associated with several measures of pregnancy outcome, the predictive power of alcohol consumption in relation to more rigorously defined birth abnormalities was extremely small and was less than that of either previous terminations of pregnancy, history of live births, or smoking. As stated above, this suggests that alcohol only played a very minor role in relation to the fetal harm noted in this study. In addition, factor analysis indicated that there were no specific types of birth abnormalities that clustered together in concert with alcohol consumption (see pages 119–20). No obvious 'syndrome' of alcohol-related abnormalities was evident among the babies in this study group.

6 Follow-up of babies

The fourth wave of data collection was related to assessing the initial development of the surviving offspring. This was carried out between August 1981 and April 1983. A total of 835 surviving babies (82.5 per cent) of the study group were examined. The remaining 173 infants were not located, since their parents had moved or were not traced. In addition, there were four neonatal deaths.

Data were collected by examination of the babies. This was carried out by the respondents' own health visitors. This examination produced information on baby's age in weeks, weight, length, head circumference, and palpebral fissure size. Information on the babies' development was also noted, as were feeding habits, feeding difficulties, sleep patterns, and general health. (See Appendix IV for full details.)

This fourth and final wave of the study was intended to take place when these babies were approximately 12 weeks old. However, since the researcher was not informed by clinic staff of the births of all the babies as they occurred, 601 of the babies were examined between 10 and 14 weeks of age and 179 were examined after this age. In addition, information was gathered from the case notes of fifty-five babies aged younger than 10 weeks. In the cases where examination took place before 10 weeks or after 14 weeks, a check was made of the baby's weight, length, and head circumference on the development chart used by the study hospital (Gairdner and Pearson 1971). Information was then noted as to whether the baby's growth was within normal limits for age.

RESULTS

As noted above, data relating to 835 infants were obtained. Of these, 601 were aged 10–14 weeks. In addition, no information was obtained about a further 173 infants. This constitutes a net response rate of 82.5 per cent. This chapter presents information relating to the 601 respondents' infants aged 10–14 weeks. The number of alcohol-related problems exhibited by surviving offspring aged 10–14 weeks is shown in *Table 20*.

Table 20 The number of alcohol-related problems in surviving offspring

number of abnormalities	N	%
0	535	89.8
1	59	9.9
2	2	0.3

Altogether 10.2 per cent of these infants were noted as having one or more alcohol-related problems. As in the previous chapter, it is emphasized that for most children these 'problems' were trivial.

The relationship between each of the abnormalities included in the 3 month check and the 4 measures of maternal alcohol consumption collected at 3 months of pregnancy was examined.

Seven of the abnormalities were recorded in continuous measures, nine were dichotomous (yes/no). Analysis for the continuous measures was conducted by partial correlation. This simultaneously controlled for mother's age, smoking habits, consumption of legal and illicit drugs, and the occupational status of each respondent's husband, boyfriend, or cohabitee. Of the seven continuous variables thus examined, only one was significantly correlated with at least one measure of maternal drinking.

As shown by *Table 21*, poor general health was slightly but significantly correlated with maximum day's alcohol consumption during the first trimester. This correlation was extremely modest.

Analysis for the nine dichotomous variables was conducted by a two-tailed T-test. This revealed a significant difference only in relation to growth deficiency. This was slightly distinguished by three measures of alcohol consumption. This is elaborated in *Table 22*.

Since only two abnormalities appeared to be associated with maternal drinking, it was not possible to produce a 'scale' like that described in chapter 6.

Table 21 Problems at three months of age which correlated significantly with baseline alcohol consumption measures (continuous variables)

variables	total previous week's consumption	maximum day's consumption in the previous week	maximum day's consumption in first trimester of pregnancy	typical day's consumption before pregnancy
poor general health	+ 0.17*	NS	NS	NS

* $p < 0.05$

The prevalence of these two problems was examined in relation to whether or not the babies' mothers were abstainers (who had consumed no alcohol since conception), light drinkers (who had consumed between 1 and 4 units on their maximum day since conception), or heavy drinkers (who had consumed 5 units or more on their maximum drinking day since conception). As already noted, 10.2 per cent of surviving infants had one or more abnormal features. A dichotomy was made between those who had no problems and those who had one or two.

Table 23 Risk of problems at the age of 12 weeks by drinking status of mother

drinking status of mother	infants with problems	
	N	% of each sub-group
abstainers (n = 126)	10	7.9
light drinkers (n = 307)	30	9.8
heavy drinkers (n = 164)	21	12.8

(x^2 = 2.04: df = 2: NS)

Table 23 indicates that there were no significant differences between the proportions of abnormal offspring in the three sub-groups.

Table 24 Rise of infant problems by maximum day's alcohol consumption during the first trimester

maximum day's consumption during first trimester	infants with problems	
	N	% of each sub-group
no alcohol consumed (n = 126)	10	7.9
between 1 and 9 units consumed (n = 446)	45	10.1
10 units or more consumed (n = 24)	6	25.0

94 Women, Drinking, and Pregnancy

Table 22 Problem at three months of age which was significantly associated with baseline alcohol consumption (dichotomous variables)

variable	total previous week's consumption			maximum day's consumption in previous weeks			maximum day's consumption in first trimester of pregnancy		
	without probs	with probs	T value	without probs	with probs	T value	without probs	with probs	T value
growth deficiency									
$\bar{x}^a$	1.3	2.1	2.13*b	0.9	1.4	2.17*c	3.2	4.6	2.89**d
SD^a	2.6	2.8		1.6	1.8		3.1	3.1	
N	553	43		553	43		553	43	

degrees of freedom = 594 (pooled variance)
* p < 0.05   ** p < 0.01   a = units of alcohol
Note: In view of the marked skewing in distribution of alcohol consumption these measures were $\log_{10}$ converted. The results of this procedure was as follows; b t = 2.64; df = 594; p < 0.01
                              c t = 2.28; df = 594; p < 0.05
                              d t = 2.83; df = 594; p < 0.01

A higher cut-off point between 'light' and 'heavy' drinker was again adopted so that a 'heavy drinker' was one who had drunk not 5 but 10 units or more on maximum day's consumption. The number of expected values in this sub-group was too small to permit an x^2 analysis. Even so, there were differences in the risks of respondents in each of these sub-groups, producing infants with one or two problems. These are shown in *Table 24*.

Six of the twenty-four infants whose mothers drank 10 or more units on their maximum day's drinking in the first trimester had one or two problems. These 'very heavy drinkers' had a risk of such features that exceeded that of other respondents by more than twofold.

A further analysis was conducted. Once more respondents were dichotomized into those whose offspring exhibited problems and those whose did not. These sub-groups were compared in relation to their mean levels of alcohol consumption. Significant differences emerged in relation to both previous week's consumption and to maximum day's consumption in the first trimester of pregnancy. Respondents whose offspring had problems reported an average consumption of 1.4 units in the previous weeks. Others averaged 0.9 units on this occasion.

Respondents whose infants had problems were not particularly heavy drinkers. Two women had children who had two problems. The mothers had an average maximum drinking day consumption since pregnancy of only 4.5 units.

As reiterated in the previous chapter, one of the aims of this study was to ascertain whether or not infant abnormalities constituted a syndrome. A factor analysis was once more conducted. This analysis involved twenty-six variables. These were twelve 'baseline' variables related to the mother, such as alcohol and drug use, coffee and tea consumption, age, stress and occupational status of respondent's husband, cohabitee, or boyfriend. In addition, the fourteen infant problems were included.

As in chapter 5, this analysis was conducted to ascertain if any grouping of the variables had enough in common to constitute specific factors. Eleven factors emerged. As in chapter 5, no clear-cut constellation of variables was evident (for full details see Appendix V). Again, there did not appear to be any indication that specific problems were clustered with maternal alcohol- consumption data.

One of the few studies that can be used for comparison is the Seattle study where Streissguth and her colleagues followed up a cohort of 462 infants at 8 months. They found 'Infant mental and motor development at 8 months had a significant inverse relationship to maternal alcohol use during pregnancy, even after adjustment for other relevant variables, including smoking' (Little 1981: 165). Like the present study, this American investigation indicated that maternal drinking is indeed associated with some growth and development problems in the infant.

SUMMARY

As noted in chapter 5, further exploration of the data collected by the present study was conducted in an attempt to clarify the relevance of the baseline data in relation to growth and development around 12 weeks. As noted above, analysis revealed that alcohol consumption was *weakly associated* with only two several measures of growth and development. As found in the third wave of data collected on pregnancy outcome, these results suggest that alcohol only played a very minor role in relation to the abnormalities of growth and development found at 12 weeks in this study.

As will already be obvious, the analytic strategy adopted in this chapter was that used in relation to the third wave of data discussed in chapter 5. The third and fourth waves of data produced parallel and compatible results. Indeed, a remarkable level of consistency emerged that lends strength to the general conclusions derived from this study.

7 Summary and conclusions

This study had two distinguishing features. The first of these was the care with which the alcohol consumption histories were collected. The second feature was the range and variety of possible confounding factors that were taken into account.

LEVEL OF RESPONSE

A great deal of time was spent at the outset of this study both with members of the nursing administration and, more relevantly, with the midwives in the antenatal clinic. The main reason for this was to form a good relationship with the clinic staff in which the required number of women could be interviewed without disrupting the smooth running of the clinic. This, along with the fact that the researcher was a qualified nurse, and therefore understood some of the practical difficulties of imposing a research project upon a hospital setting, proved extremely successful. The low refusal rate may have been due in part to the unfamiliar setting. These women had not attended this clinic before during their current pregnancy and were perhaps reluctant to refuse to participate. The other main factor involved the choice and training of interviewers. Clearly, using interviewers who were not clinic staff members is only possible or indeed desirable during a study of this kind. It could not be done as a routine part of the obstetric case-taking procedure. It is important to note that asking questions about topics that are seen as intimate or sensitive is a skill and should be taught, not left to chance, as it often is in the nursing and medical profession.

VALIDITY

Surveys of drinking behaviour are notorious for producing distorted results. However, the interviewers mainly felt the respondents enjoyed the interview, seemed quite relaxed in a confidential setting, and not at all concerned about answering questions honestly on their drinking and other topics. The respondents were interviewed if possible just before seeing the obstetrician; this left little time for them to discuss the interview with each other and helped to prevent contamination. It is possible that the clinic was a stressful setting for data collection. It would have been useful to have interviewed a sub-sample of women in their own homes. Unfortunately, this was not feasible due to financial and time constraints.

RESULTS

The primary aim of this study was to establish whether or not birth abnormalities were associated with self-reported rates of drinking by pregnant women. As can be seen from *Tables 13, 14* and *15* a number of birth abnormalities and perinatal difficulties were individually significantly associated with baseline alcohol consumption measures. Having established an association, two secondary aims were pursued: to ascertain at what levels of alcohol consumption, birth damage is evident; and to investigate whether or not evident alcohol related birth damage does constitute a syndrome.

The first of these two aims was examined by comparing three sub-groups of respondents. These were: abstainers, those who had not drunk during pregnancy; light drinkers, those who had drunk between one and four units on the maximum drinking day since conception and heavy drinkers, those respondents who had consumed over four units of alcohol on the maximum drinking day since conception.

As noted in chapters 5 and 6, the results showed that the offspring of the heavy drinkers were not *significantly* more likely to have abnormalities or problems than were babies of women in the abstainers or light-drinkers sub-groups. Even so, heavy drinkers did have an increased risk of producing damaged babies. Women whose maximum day's alcohol consumption during the first trimester had exceeded 10 units were significantly more likely than other respondents to have produced babies with two or more abnormalities. This is shown in *Table 17*. In addition, this sub-group of heavy-drinking women had a risk of one or two infant problems (at 12 weeks of age), which was double that of other respondents. This is shown in *Table 24*. However, the list of infant abnormalities used in this study included many minor perinatal problems such as mild jaundice and lower birth weight. The reasons for these problems are many, and an association with alcohol is probably no more relevant than the association with some of the mothers' dietary habits. The most important part of the analysis was the use of stepwise multiple regression. This analysis was conducted in an attempt to clarify the strength of alcohol as a cause of fetal harm. As noted in chapter 6 alcohol was not strongly predictive; indeed, the drugs that accounted for the greatest variance in the multiple regressions were tobacco and illegal drugs (see *Table 21*).

Heavy drinkers in this study were more at risk of producing damaged babies, but it was something other than their alcohol consumption that caused the damage. In several studies heavy drinking has been associated with tobacco and other drug use, increased maternal age, parity, stress, and with unmarried motherhood (Abel 1982; Weiner *et. al.* 1983; Rosett and Weiner 1984). In time, other relevant factors will probably be identified.

The issue of the relationship of low birth weight to alcohol consumption is now well documented; this study, in agreement with many others, again showed an association between reduced birth weight and alcohol consumption. However, if Baird's work in 1974 is taken into account, the birth weight, not only of the baby but also of its mother, needs to be known. As far as this author knows, no study into drinking in pregnancy has taken this latter factor into account.

The second of the two aims noted above, whether or not alcohol-related birth damage does constitute a syndrome, produced an equally negative conclusion in this study. The clear cluster of features that reputedly constitute the fetal alcohol syndrome was notably absent. However, the levels of alcohol consumption were relatively low in this particular study group.

CONCLUSIONS

The results of this study show that birth abnormalities were slightly *associated* with but not caused by maternal alcohol consumption. Very heavy drinkers (those consuming 10 units or more at one time in the first trimester) were significantly more likely to produce babies with abnormalities than were either light drinkers or abstainers. However, after controlling for a number of confounding variables, alcohol consumption recorded during the first phase of this study did not emerge as a substantial predictor of this fetal harm. This conclusion is extremely important. The results of this study do not support the clear claims of some earlier workers (for example, Streissguth *et al.*) that moderate alcohol consumption in pregnancy is a *cause* of fetal harm.

It is emphasized that this study related to a group of 'normal women'. The overwhelming majority of these individuals were not heavy drinkers or dependent on alcohol. These results do not form a basis for generalizing about heavy-drinking women in relation to whom quite different conclusions might be reached. Alcohol-related harm does not have a simple linear relationship with alcohol consumption. Fetal damage too may be exponentially related to maternal drinking. This link may only be apparent amongst much heavier drinkers than the women in this study.

The main drug predictor of fetal harm in this study were tobaccos and illegal drugs. This is consistent with other evidence. In 1980 the United States Surgeon General noted in a report entitled *The Health Consequences of Smoking for Women* that: 'The risk of spontaneous abortion, fetal death and neo-natal death increases directly with increasing levels of maternal smoking during pregnancy'.

It must be a cause for concern that fewer than 30 per cent of smokers in this study stopped smoking when they became aware of their pregnancy.

IMPLICATIONS OF RESULTS

The issue of assessing 'risk' in relation to drinking during pregnancy is of great importance. In trying to assess risk in the laboratory or round the 'decision-making' table it is all too easy to forget some of the less tangible factors. Weighing such questions as 'how safe is safe?' or 'what is an acceptable level of risk?' inevitably means that decisions have to be made.

It is irresponsible, patronizing, and dangerous to assume that pregnant women need to be 'protected' from information pertaining to themselves or their babies. Uninformed half-truths and exaggerated statements are frequently made on the subject of drinking in pregnancy. This is all the more reason why professionals caring for such women should be informed about developments in the research field.

However, as Fischhoff *et al.* in their useful book *Acceptable Risk* go on to say: 'All formal analysis relies on the strong behavioral assumptions whose common element is that decision makers are highly rational, sensitive to limits of their own knowledge and ready to ask for help when it is needed' (1983: 114). It is worrying to note that the many dogmatic and extremist statements quoted in chapter 1 clearly show that this is a risky assumption. We should not wait till the ideal piece of research has been conducted, which proves conclusively one way or the other, before making the concern public. It is nothing more than responsible, caring behaviour. However, as Fischhoff *et al.* also state:

'The simplifying assumptions and deficiencies of even the best analysis render them only an *aid* to decision making. In this view, the goal of analysis is to clarify a problem's facts, values, and uncertainties, thereby making it easier for decision makers to rely on their own intuitions in choosing an alternative.'

(Fischhoff *et al.* 1983: 101)

RECOMMENDATIONS

FUTURE RESEARCH

It is known that women taking hormone supplements experience a decrease in the rate of ethanol metabolism, and that the blood alcohol levels of women differ at different times in the menstrual cycle (Jones and Jones 1976). Given the massive shifts in hormone levels at conception and later in pregnancy and the inconsistency of this in different individuals, the possibility of blood alcohol peaking at far higher levels than have been measured up till now is possible. Concern over pollution and the increase in additives both to water and food has been growing from about the time that most recent concern over fetal alcohol effects have been voiced. In some areas, like Edinburgh where this study was conducted, there is a high level of lead found in the water. Such levels have been shown to cause retardation. Much more time and effort has to be spent on teasing out these different issues.

There are many uncertainties left in this area. Could a combination of alcohol and acetaldehyde at higher levels of consumption cause harm? Does history of alcohol abuse in parents affect sensitivity in their offspring? It is now known that children of parents with a drink problem have higher acetaldehyde levels for the same amount of alcohol as do children of non-problem drinking parents (Schukitt 1980). It is known that Thalidomide, for instance, only caused severe harm if taken between the fifth and ninth week of pregnancy (Knightly *et al.* 1979). Is there a possibility of there being 'windows' in the pregnancy when alcohol in combination with other factors can cause harm?

The present study must obviously be replicated. A larger sample size would be an improvement. Future studies in this field could usefully follow up the childhood development of the offspring of a group of women who drank heavily during pregnancy. This type of approach has been adopted by Streissguth *et al.* (1980). Adapting the methods of the present study, such heavy drinkers could be identified at follow-up, together with a control group of light drinkers. This would aid the assessment of more subtle or longer-term problems such as behavioural and school-related difficulties. It would also allow for testing of such things as blood acetaldehyde levels in older children. This may throw more light on whether acetaldehyde levels in the children of the heavy drinkers differ from those of the light drinkers. In the present study 9 per cent of fathers and 2 per cent of mothers of the respondents had experienced problems with their drinking. This may mean that information on parental drinking might highlight alcohol/acetaldehyde sensitivities in the children when they reach childbearing age. Work is being conducted on genetic susceptibilities. Information on parental alcohol consumption might be useful in this context. This issue of dose response versus threshold effect may be clarified in future with the help of trend analysis.

TRAINING OF HEALTH PROFESSIONALS

All initial antenatal clinic assessment should contain information on drinking problems. Information on maximum day's consumption since last menstrual period may be a useful marker. Health staff involved in caring for women who attend family planning clinics, preconceptual clinics, and antenatal clinics should be aware of the conflicting information available on the possible risks of drinking in pregnancy and standard, consistent messages should be given. The view of this author is as follows: according to the results of this study and a number of others (see chapter 1), alcohol in moderate doses does *not* appear to cause harm. This should be followed with the provision of an indication of what constitutes 'moderate' drinking. In this study this would be one or two units once or twice a week.

HEALTH EDUCATION

The results of this study are broadly consistent with those of earlier prospective investigations in this field. It is remarkable therefore that some of the earlier results have been interpreted to support the view that moderate alcohol consumption in pregnancy is a substantial cause for concern. In some countries, particularly the United States, this topic is now the subject of a highly publicized, and sometimes highly charged, debate.

At the present time and with available knowledge, statements about moderate drinking in pregnancy should not be alarmist. Statements about the role of tobacco, however, should be more emphatic. Finally, care should be taken that this important subject is not taken out of context and used in the emotive way that colours many of the pronouncements heard in the alcohol field.

Appendix I
Wave one interview schedules

During the first wave of data collection, two instruments were used. The first of these, an interview schedule, is presented in Appendix I(a). This was used to collect information from mothers at the booking-in clinic and was administered by trained interviewers. The second instrument, presented in Appendix I(b), relates to information extracted from mothers' clinic case notes.

(a) THE INITIAL INTERVIEW

All 1,008 respondents were initially interviewed using a twenty-one-page schedule. For the sake of brevity, this appendix simply lists the questions included in the document.

1. Are you:
   Married?
   Living with someone?
   Single?
   Living apart/separated?
   Divorced?
   Other?
2. In which country were you born?
3. What is your occupation?
4. What is your husband's/boyfriend's occupation?
5. What was your husband's/boyfriend's last job (if unemployed)?
6. What height is your husband/boyfriend?
7. Have you been in contact with German measles (rubella) within the last 12 weeks?

8. How many people live in your household?
9. How many rooms does your household have?
10. Do you ever drink alcohol?
11. When was the last time you had a drink?
12a How many days a week do you usually have a drink?
12b *If 'nil'*: how often do you have a drink?
13. How much do you drink on a typical drinking day?
14. How often did you drink before pregnancy?
15. How much did you drink on a typical drinking day before pregnancy?
16. What have you had to drink over the past 7 days?
17a Was that typical of what you have been drinking lately?
17b *If answer was 'no'*: Was that more or less than usual?
18a Since becoming pregnant have you drunk more or less alcohol than before pregnancy or has your alcohol consumption remained about the same?
18b *If answer is 'more' or 'less'*: Why do you think this change has occurred?
19. Since becoming pregnant have you noticed any change in the effect alcohol has on you?
20. What was this change in effect?
21. During the past 12 weeks have you ever been merry, happy or intoxicated due to drinking?
22. How many times in the past 12 weeks have you felt like this?
23. What is the most alcohol you have drunk on any one day in the past 12 weeks?
24a Does your husband/boyfriend drink alcohol?
24b *If 'yes'*: Has his drinking caused any problems at work, in his health or in the family?
25. What was this?
26a Does/did your father/stepfather drink alcohol?
26b *If 'yes'*: Has his drinking caused any problems at work, in his health or in the family?
27a Does/did your mother/stepmother drink alcohol?
27b *If 'yes'*: Has her drinking caused any problems at work, in her health or in the family?
28. Have you ever had any of the following?
    Inflamed stomach (gastritis)
    Stomach ulcer
    Liver trouble/jaundice
    Peripheral neuritis (pain and tingling in hands and feet for

more than 2 hours at a time)
Kidney trouble
Heart condition
Chest condition
Diabetes
Recurrent urinary infection
Gynaecological problems

29. Have you ever been worried about your drinking?
30a Has your drinking ever caused you any problems?
30b *If 'yes'*: What were these problems?
31. Have you ever felt you should cut down on your drinking?
32. Have you ever sought professional help or advice because of your drinking?
33. Do you smoke?
34. Did you smoke before pregnancy and stop when you found out you were pregnant?
35. What do you mainly smoke?
36. How many cigarettes/cigars do you smoke in a day?
37. How much tobacco do you smoke in a week?
38a Since becoming pregnant do you smoke more or less than before or has your smoking remained the same?
38b *If 'more' or 'less'*: Why do you think this change has occurred?
39a Have you been under any emotional stress within the past 12 weeks?
39b *If 'yes'*: Could you tell me what this was?
40a Have you ever had trouble with your nerves?
40b *If 'yes'*: Could you tell me what this was?
41. Have you ever sought medical advice or help for this problem?
42. Have you ever taken an overdose?
43. Would you tell me if you have taken any of the following medication during the last 12 weeks?
    Analgesics (e.g. Aspirin)
    Antacids (e.g. Mucaine)
    Laxatives (e.g. Senokot)
    Antibiotics (e.g. Penicillin, Septrin)
    Tranquillisers (e.g. Valium)
    Barbiturates (e.g. Phenobarbitone)
    Hypnotics (e.g. sleeping tablets)
    Anti-epileptic (e.g. Epanutin, Mysolin)
    Anti-nausea (e.g. Debendox)
    Any other

44. Can you tell me if you have taken any of the following drugs during the last 12 weeks?
    Cannabis (marihuana, pot)
    Amphetamines (speed)
    L.S.D.
    Opium
    Morphine
    Heroin
    Glues or solvents
    Any other
45. How many cups of coffee do you drink in a day?
46. How many cups of tea do you drink in a day?
47. Do you take three meals each day?
48. Which meal is most often missed?
49. Is your appetite usually good?
50a Since becoming pregnant are you eating more, less or about the same as you were before?
50b *If 'less'*: why is this?
51. How often do you eat beef or lamb, pork, or poultry?
52. How often do you eat fish?
53. How often do you eat liver?
54. How often do you eat eggs?
55. How much milk do you drink daily?
56. Do you take any of these foods at least two to three times a week?
    Wholemeal bread
    Ryvita or similar
    Cornflakes, Rice Crispies
    Wheat germ
57. How often do you eat fresh fruit?
58. How often do you eat fresh vegetables?
59. Do you take any vitamin supplements?
60. *If yes*: what are these?

At the end of this interview the respondent was asked whether or not she would be willing to be re-interviewed four months later.

(b) THE INITIAL CLINICAL RECORD

Information from all 1,008 respondents' clinic case notes was extracted using a twelve page schedule. The topics included in this instrument are listed below.

1. Age
2. Height
3. Weight
4. Blood pressure
5. Result of urine testing
6. Number of weeks pregnant
7. Number of previous pregnancies
8. Number of live births
9. Any multiple births (twins, triplets)
10. Number of stillbirths
11. Number of spontaneous abortions (miscarriages)
12. Number of terminations of pregnancy
13. Number of children with physical handicap
14. Place in family of child/children with a physical handicap
15. Full description of each child's physical handicap
16. Number of children mildly physically handicapped
17. Number of children moderately physically handicapped
18. Number of children severely physically handicapped
19. Number of children with mental handicap
20. Place in family of child/children with mental handicap
21. Full description of each child's mental handicap
22. Number of children with mild mental handicap
23. Number of children with moderate mental handicap
24. Number of children with severe mental handicap
25. Results of Blood Test MCV
26. Results of Blood Test Gamma GT

Appendix II
Wave two interview schedules

During the follow-up of the three sub-groups of respondents (abstainers, light, and heavy drinkers) the following shortened and amended instruments were used. Again, the first of these, presented in Appendix IIa, was used to collect information from mothers at their 34-week examination and was administered by trained interviewers. The second instrument, presented in Appendix IIb, relates to information extracted from mothers' clinic case notes.

(a) THE FOLLOW-UP INTERVIEW

All 255 respondents included in the second wave of data collection were interviewed using a standardized schedule of fourteen pages. The contents are summarized below.

1a Do you ever drink alcohol?

1b *If 'yes'*: since becoming pregnant, have you drunk more or less alcohol than before pregnancy or has your alcohol consumption remained about the same?

1c *If 'more' or 'less'*: why do you think this change has occurred?

2. When was the last time you had a drink?

3. How many days a week do you usually have a drink?

4. Please tell me exactly what you had to drink over the past 7 days.

5a Was that typical of what you have been drinking lately?

5b *If 'no'*: was that more or less than usual?

6a Has your alcohol consumption changed during the last 4 months?

6b *If 'yes'*: are you drinking more or less?

7. Why do you think this change has occurred?
8a During the past 4 months have you ever been merry, happy or intoxicated due to drinking?
8b *If 'yes'*: How many times in the past 4 months have you felt like this?
9. What is the most alcohol you have drunk on any one day in the past four months?
10. Do you smoke?
11a *If 'yes'*: Have you smoked throughout your pregnancy?
11b *If 'no'*: When did you restart smoking?
12. What do you mainly smoke?
13. How many cigarettes/cigars do you smoke in a day?
14. How much tobacco do you smoke in a week? (if respondent rolls her own cigarettes)?
15a Have you been under any 'emotional stress' within the past 4 months?
15b *If 'yes'*: Could you tell me what this was?
16. Would you tell me if you have taken any of the following medicines during the last four months?
    Analgesics (e.g. Aspirin)
    Antacids (e.g. Mucaine)
    Laxatives (e.g. Senokot)
    Antibiotics (e.g. Penicillin, Septrin)
    Tranquillisers (e.g. Valium)
    Barbiturates (e.g. Pheno-barb)
    Hypnotics (e.g. sleeping tablets)
    Anti-epileptic (e.g. Epanutin, Mysolin)
    Anti-nausea (e.g. Debendox)
    Any other
17a Have you taken any other medicines during the last 4 months?
17b *If 'yes'*: what was this?
18. Can you tell me if you have taken any of the following drugs during the last 4 months?
    Cannabis (marihuana, pot)
    Amphetamines (speed)
    L.S.D.
    Opium
    Morphine
    Heroin
    Glues or solvents
    Any other

19. How many cups of coffee do you drink in a day?
20. How many cups of tea do you drink in a day?
21a Do you take three meals each day?
21b *If answer is 'no'*: Which meal is most often missed?
22. Is your appetite usually good?
23. How often do you eat beef or lamb, pork or poultry?
24. How often do you eat fish?
25. How often do you eat liver?
26. How often do you eat eggs?
27. How much milk do you drink daily?
28. Do you take any of these foods at least two to three times a week?
    Wholemeal bread
    Ryvita or similar
    Cornflakes, Rice Crispies
    Wheat germ
29. How often do you eat fresh fruit?
30. How often do you eat fresh vegetables?
31a Do you take any vitamin supplements?
31b *If 'yes'*: what are these?
32. Are you taking your iron/folic acid tablets regularly?

(b) THE FOLLOW-UP CLINICAL RECORD

The following information from the 255 respondents re-interviewed during phase two of this study was derived from clinic case notes and recorded in a four page instrument.
1. Weight
2. Blood pressure
3. Result of urine testing
4a Has patient been admitted at any time during this pregnancy?
4b *If 'yes'*: Number of admissions
5. Reason for admissions
6. Any infections during this pregnancy (record any infections fully)
7. Any other problems during this pregnancy which did not require admission (record any other problems fully)
8. Results of Blood Test MCV
9. Results of Blood Test Gamma GT

Appendix III
Wave three examination schedules

Information was extracted from the clinic case notes of all live births produced by the study group. This information was collected using a five-page schedule. The items included in this instrument are listed below.

1. Maternal record
2. Drugs taken in pregnancy
3. Gestation at administration of drug
4. Amniocentesis
5. Labour record
      Onset
      Fetal distress
      Drugs given in labour
      Type of delivery
      Complications of delivery
      Placental weight
      Placental condition
6. Birth record
      Gestation
      Membrane rupture/delivery interval
      Date of birth
      Agpar score 1 minute and 5 minutes
      Resuscitation
      Birth weight
      Whether singleton, twin, or triplet
      Sex
      Occipito-frontal head circumference on the third day
      Length

Number of umbilical vessels
Gestational age by assessment of baby by scoring method
Transfers (e.g. special nursery)
State of:
  head
  face
  eyes
  ears
  nose
  mouth
  palate
  neck
  skin
  umbilicus
  c.v.s. femoral pulses
  heart sounds
  murmurs
  chest auscultation
  abdomen
  spleen
  liver
  kidneys
  genitalia
  anus
  spine
  arms
  hands
  legs
  feet
  hips
  posture and movement
  muscle tone
  grasp
  moro reflex
  cry
Palpebral fissure length
Jaundice
Absence or presence of:
  infection
  significant hypotonia
  cyanosis (central)

oedema
convulsions
recurrent apnoea
assisted ventilation after 30 minutes
feeding difficulty
vomiting
diarrhoea
Feeding
  breast
  bottle
  breast and cup
  other
General condition
Discharge, e.g. Home
              Residential or Foster Care

Appendix IV
Wave four
examination schedules

During the fourth wave of data collection the surviving offspring were examined at the age of 12 weeks. This examination was carried out by the mothers' and babies' own health visitor. The information elicited was recorded in a two page instrument and is listed below.

 1. Mother's name
 2. Mother's date of birth
 3. Date of examination
 4. Baby's name
 5. Sex of baby
 6. Baby's age in weeks
 7. Baby's weight
 8. Baby's length
 9. Baby's head circumference
10. Palpebral fissure size
11. Development chart
       lifted prone, holds head up
       lying prone, lifts head 45–90 per cent
       pull to sit, only slight head lag
       holds rattle momentarily
       supine, watches own hands
       follows object from side to side
       squeals of pleasure
12. Type of feeding
13. Feeding problems
14. Sleeping
15. General health

Appendix V
Supplementary
analysis from waves
three and four

One of the aims of this study was to ascertain whether or not birth abnormalities constituted a syndrome. In order to investigate this a factor analysis was conducted. A factor can be loosely defined as the outcome of discovering a group of variables having a certain characteristic. This analysis involved forty-nine variables. These included nineteen types of birth abnormalities, seventeen difficulties in the perinatal period and thirteen variables related to the mother. Those relating to birth abnormalities and perinatal difficulties had each been noted in three or more of the babies in the study. Variables relating to fewer infants were excluded. The thirteen variables relating to the mother included baseline data, such as maximum alcohol consumption in one day in the previous week, maximum day's consumption in the first trimester, typical drinking day's consumption before pregnancy, smoking, and other drug use. Only three of the sixteen factors that emerged had any obvious clusters of features above the r = 0.6 level. These are shown in *Table AI*.

As can be seen from *Table AI*, these factors showed obvious clusters:

factor 1 – severe respiratory difficulties plus three abnormalities
factor 2 – resuscitation problems
factor 3 – alcohol consumption

Table A1 Factor analysis: factors involving obvious clusters

variable	Factor number		
	1	3	4
severe respiratory difficulties factor (1)			
central cyanosis	+ 0.73		
convulsions	+ 0.80		
recurrent apnoea	+ 0.81		
assisted ventilation after 30 minutes	+ 0.64		
vomiting	+ 0.81		
diarrhoea	+ 0.81		
abnormalities of:-			
palate	+ 0.77		
legs	+ 0.91		
femoral pulses	+ 0.72		
resuscitation factor (3)			
resuscitation		+ 0.81	
Apgar score at 1 minute		+ 0.85	
Apgar score at 2 minutes		+ 0.71	
alcohol consumption factor (4)			
maximum day's consumption in the previous week			+ 0.71
maximum day's consumption in the past 12 weeks			+ 0.79
typical drinking day before pregnancy			+ 0.68

NOTE Factor 1 explained 15.4 per cent of the variables (Eigenvalue = 7.5)

Factors 1 and 2 are obvious clusters but are not grouped with any alcohol consumption measures. Conversely, factor 3 clusters the peak alcohol consumption measures during pregnancy with typical day's drinking prior to pregnancy but not with fetal harm. There is no indication that specific birth abnormalities cluster with maternal alcohol consumption data.

SUPPLEMENTARY ANALYSIS WAVE FOUR

This factor analysis was conducted in an attempt to assess whether growth, developmental or general problems, for example, sleeping or feeding difficulties at 12 weeks, were clustered with baseline alcohol consumption measures. This analysis involved four growth measures, seven developmental measures and twelve maternal baseline data measures. The twelve maternal variables included maximum day's alcohol consumption in the previous week, maximum day's alcohol consumption in the first trimester, typical day's drinking before pregnancy, smoking, occupational status of husband/boyfriend or cohabitee, and other drug use. Only two of the eleven factors that emerged had any obvious clusters of features above the r = 0.6 level. These are shown in *Table A2.*

Table A2   Factor analysis: factors involving obvious clusters

variable	factor number	
	1	2
alcohol consumption factor (1)		
maximum day's consumption in the previous week	+ 0.68	
maximum day's consumption in the first trimester	+ 0.78	
typical day's drinking before pregnancy	+ 0.68	
developmental factor (2)		
lifted prone, holds head up		+ 0.79
lying prone, lifts head 45–90%		+ 0.74
pull to sit, only slight head lag		+ 0.71

NOTE Factor 1 explained 9.2 per cent of the variance (Eigenvalue = 2.4)

As can be seen from *Table A2*, these factors showed obvious clusters:-

factor 1 – alcohol consumption
factor 2 – developmental variables.

As in the factor analysis conducted on the data from wave three, there is no indication that specific growth or developmental variables clustered with any maternal baseline variables.

Taken together, these factors show that although the alcohol consumption variables cluster together, there is no indication that infant problems are present in the same group.

This analysis did not indicate any obvious clustering of alcohol consumption measure and abnormalities either at birth or at 12 weeks of age. However, it must be emphasized that the respondents in this study group were overwhelmingly moderate drinkers. These results do not form a basis for generalization about heavy or dependent drinkers.

Bibliography

This bibliography lists the references that were used in the compilation of this book. Not all have been directly cited in the text.

Abel, E. L. (1979) Sex Ratio in FAS. *Lancet* 2: 105.

—— (1980) The Fetal Alcohol Syndrome: Behavioral Teratology. *Psychological Bulletin* 87: 29–50.

—— (1981) Behavioral Teratology of Alcohol. *Psychological Bulletin* 90 (3): 564–81.

—— (1981) *Fetal Alcohol Syndrome vol. 1: An Annotated and Comprehensive Bibliography.* Florida: CRC Press.

—— (1981) *Fetal Alcohol Syndrome vol. 2: Human Studies.* Florida: CRC Press.

—— (ed.) (1982) *Fetal Alcohol Syndrome vol. 3: Animal Studies.* Florida: CRC Press.

—— (1982) *Alcohol and Reproduction. A Bibliography.* Connecticut: Greenwood Press.

—— (1982) Characteristics of Mothers of Fetal Alcohol Syndrome Children. *Neurobehavioral Toxicology and Teratology* 3: 3–4.

—— (1982) Consumption of Alcohol during Pregnancy: A Review of Effects on Growth and Development of Offspring. *Human Biology* 54 (3): 421–53.

Abramson, J. H. (1984) *Survey Methods in Community Medicine.* Edinburgh: Churchill Livingstone.

Addendum (1982) Alcohol and Alcoholism. *Bulletin* of *British Journal of Psychiatry* April: 69.

Alderson, M. (1976) *An Introduction to Epidemiology.* London: Macmillan.

Aldred, C. (1981) *Women at Work.* London: Pan Books.

Alfawap Journal (1977) Pregnant Women Shouldn't Drink At All. *The Journal* 1 December: 60. (Full edition given over to fetal alcohol syndrome issues.)

—— (1981) *Should I Drink?* London: Health education pamphlet. Handicapped Children Fund.

Alpert, J. J., Day, N., Dooling, E., Hingson, R., Oppenheimer, E., Rosett, H. L., Weiner, L., and Zuckerman, B. (1981) Maternal Alcohol Consumption and Newborn Assessment: Methodology of the Boston City Hospital Prospective Study. *Neurobehavioral Toxicology and Teratology* **3**: 195–201.

Altman, B. (1976) Fetal Alcohol Syndrome. *Journal of Pediatric Ophthalmology* **13**: 255.

Anon (1942) Effects of Single Large Alcohol Intake on the Fetus (Queries and Minor Notes). *Journal of the American Medical Association* **120**: 88.

—— (1947) Alcohol, Heredity and Germ Damage. *Quarterly Journal Studies on Alcohol* Supplement 5.

—— (1949) Effects of Alcohol and Tobacco on Fertility. *British Medical Journal* **2**: 768.

—— (1954) Smoking and Drinking During Pregnancy (Queries and Minor Notes). *Journal of the American Medical Association* **154**: 186.

—— (1971) Alcoholic Mothers' Babies' Failure to Thrive. *Journal of the American Medical Association* **213**: 1429.

—— (1975) Bottle Babies. *Listen*: May.

—— (1975) Paediatricians Finding Fetal Alcohol Effects. *United States Medicine* 15.

—— (1975) Study Shows Rise in Drunk Newborns. *Jet Magazine* 29 May.

—— (1976) Heart Defects Accompany FAS (Medical News). *Journal of the American Medical Association* **235**: 1073.

—— (1977) Even Moderate Drinking may be Hazardous to Maturing Fetus. *Journal of the American Medical Association* **237**: 2585.

—— (1977) Fetal Alcohol Syndrome. *Food and Drug Administration Drug Bulletin* **7**: 18.

—— (1977) The FAS: a Threat to our Children. *The Globe: An International Magazine on Alcohol and Drug Problems* **2**: 3.

—— (1977) The FAS: Recent German Investigations. *The Globe: An International Magazine on Alcohol and Drug Problems* **2** (5): 22.

—— (1977) The Spectre of Fetal Alcoholism. *Emergency Medicine* **9**: 121.

—— (1978) Fetal Alcohol Syndrome. *Current Health* **2**: 12.

—— (1978) Can Alcoholic Fathers Cause Birth Defects? *Listen* March: 3.

—— (1978) Effects of Alcohol on the Fetus (letter). *New England Journal of Medicine* **298**: 55.

—— (1978) Fetal Alcohol Syndrome: New Perspectives. *Alcohol Health and Research World* **2**: 2.

—— (1978) Maternal Alcohol Consumption and Birth Weight. *British Medical Journal* **2**: 76.

—— (1978) Preventing the Birth of a Handicapped Child? *Midwives Chronicle* **91**: 34.

—— (1978) *Smoking, Drinking and Pregnancy*. Do It Now Foundation.

Institute for Chemical Survival, Phoenix, Arizona.
—— (1979) Broad Education Program on Drinking and Pregnancy. *Discus Newsletter* 384.
—— (1979) Physicians Sent Advisory on Drinking, Pregnancy. *Discus Newsletter* 386.
—— (1979) March of Dimes Joins Educational Efforts. *Discus Newsletter* 386.
—— (1979) Scientists Study FAS. *Alcoholism Newsletter* 1: 1.
—— (1980) Alcohol and Spontaneous Abortion. *Lancet* July: 26.
Anton, G. (1901) Alkoholismus und Erblichkeit (Alcoholism and Nausea). *Psychol. Wochenschr.* 14: 143.
—— (1914) Verschlechterung der Erblichkeit bei Trunkern (Worsening of Nausea in Drinkers). *Die Alkoholtrage* (Berlin) 11: 242.
Apgar, V. (1964) Drugs in Pregnancy. *Journal of the American Medical Association* 190: 840.
Apley, J. (1979) *Paediatrics: Second Edition*. London: Baillière Tindall.
Archer, J. and Lloyd, B. (1982) *Sex and Gender*. Harmondsworth: Pelican Books.
Ardener, S. (ed.) (1978) *Defining Females: The Nature of Women in Society*. London: Croom Helm.
Arlitt, A. H. and Wells, H. G. (1917) The Effect of Alcohol on Reproductive Tissues. *Journal of Experimental Medicine* 26: 769.
Arnaudova, R. and Kacvulov, A. (1978) Kafe i Bremennost (Coffee and Pregnancy). *Akush Ginekol (Moscow)* 17: 57.
Aro, T. (1983) Maternal Diseases, Alcohol Consumption and Smoking in Pregnancy Associated with Reduction Limb Defects. *Early Human Development* 9 December (1): 49–57.
Arrive, R. (1899) 'Influence de l'Alcoolisme sur le Depopulation' ('Influence of Alcoholism on Depopulation'). Thesis: University of Paris.
Arulanantham, K. and Goldstein, G. (1979) Neural Tube Defects with Fetal Alcohol Syndrome – Reply. *Journal of Pediatrics* 95: 329.
Ashley, M. J. (1979) Drinking by Mothers-to-be: A Discussion for Public Health Professionals. *Information Review* (Toronto) p. 1.
—— (1981) Alcohol Use during Pregnancy: A Challenge for the '80s. *Canadian Medical Association Journal* 125 (2): 141–43.
Asker, R. L. and Renwick, J. H. (1982) Erythrocyte Volume as a Crude Indicator of Ethanol Consumption in Pregnancy. *Clinical and Laboratory Haematology* 4 (3): 327–29.
Atkin, C. and Block, M. (1984) Content and Effects of Alcohol Advertising: A Reply to Strickland. *Journal of Studies on Alcohol* January 45 (1): 93–100.
Badinter, E. (1981) *The Myth of Motherhood: An Historical View of the Maternal Instinct*. London: Souvenir Press Ltd.
Baldwin V. J., Macleod, P. M., and Benirschke, K. (1982) Placental Findings in Alcohol Abuse in Pregnancy. *Birth Defects*: Original Article

Series **18** (3A): 89–94.

Ballantyne, J. W. (1904) *Manual of Antenatal Pathology and Hygiene: The Embryo*. Edinburgh: William Green.

—— (1917) Alcohol and Antenatal Child Welfare. *British Journal of Inebriety* **14**: 93.

Baly, M. E. (1982) *Nursing and Social Change*. London: William Heinemann.

Bancroft, J. (1983) *Human Sexuality and its Problems*. Edinburgh: Churchill Livingstone.

Banks, O. (1981) *Faces of Feminism*. Oxford: Martin Robertson.

Bardwick, J. M. (1980) *Women in Transition*. Sussex: Harvester Press.

Baric, L. and MacArthur, C. (1977) Health Norms in Pregnancy. *British Journal of Preventative and Social Medicine* **31**: 30.

Baric, L., MacArthur, C., and Sherwood, M. (1976) A Study of Health Education Aspects of Smoking in Pregnancy. *International Journal Health Education* **19**: 1.

Bark, N. (1979) Fertility and Offspring of Alcoholic Women: An Unsuccessful Search for the FAS. *British Journal of Addiction* **74**: 43.

Barker, D. J. P. and Rose, G. (1984) *Epidemiology in Medical Practice*. Edinburgh: Churchill Livingstone.

Barnes, F. H. (1915) Heredity in Alcoholism. *Long Island Medical Journal* **9**: 337.

Barr, C. L., Fountain, A. W., and Staats, W. D. (1977) Student Drug Use and Alcohol Opinionnaire and Usage Survey, Grades 6, 7, 8, 9, 10, 11, 12. Supervision of Instructional Material, Dural County Board School, Jacksonville, Florida.

Barr, H. M., Streissguth, A. P., Martin, D. C., and Horst, T. E. (1981) Methodological Issues in Assessment of Caffeine Intake: A Method for Quantifying Consumption and a Test Retest Reliability Study. In L. F. Soyka and G. P. Redmond (eds) *Drug Metabolism in the Immature Human*. New York: Raven Press.

Barrada, M. I., Virnig, N. L., Edwards, L. L., and Hakanson, E. Y. (1977) Maternal Intravenous Ethanol in the Prevention of Respiratory Distress Syndrome. *American Journal of Obstetrics and Gynecology* **129**: 25–30.

Barrison, I. G., Viola, L., and Murray-Lyon, I. M. (1980) Do Housemen Take an Adequate Drinking History? *British Medical Journal* **2**: 1040–41.

Barrison, I. G., Sampson, B., Wright, J. T., and Murray-Lyon, I. M. (1981) Are GGT and MCV Useful Markers of Excessive Drinking among Pregnant Women? *British Society of Gastroenterology* **22**: 899.

Barrison, I. G., Wright, J. T., Sampson, B., Morris, N. F., and Murray-Lyon, I. M. (1982) Screening for Alcohol Abuse in Pregnancy. *British Medical Journal* **285**: 1318–320.

Barrison, I. G., Wright, J. T., Murray-Lyon, I. M. (1983) The Hazards of Moderate Drinking During Pregnancy. *British Journal of Alcohol and Alcoholism* **16** (4): 188–99.

Barry, R. G. G. and O'Nuallan, S. O. (1975) Case Report: Foetal Alcoholism. *Irish Journal of Medical Science* 144: 286.

Barthelmess, A. (1970) Mutagenic Substances in the Human Environment. In F. Vogel and G. Rohtorn (eds) *Chemical Mutagenesis in Mammals and Man*. New York: Springer-Verlag.

Bartle, W. R., and Paton, T. W. (1978) Effects of Drugs During Pregnancy. *Moderne Medicine Canada* 33: 30.

Beattie, J. O. Day, R. E., Cockburn, F., and Garg, R. A. (1983) Alcohol and the Fetus in the West of Scotland. *British Medical Journal* 287: 17–20.

Beaumont, T. (1841–42) Remarks Made in Opposition to the Views of Dr Clutterbuck. *Lancet* 2: 340–43.

Beecher, L. (1827) *Six Sermons on the Nature, Occasions, Signs, Evils and Remedy of Intemperance*. Boston: Crocker and Brewster.

Behar, D., Berg, C. J., Rapport, J. L., Nelson, W., Linnoila, M., Cohen, M., Bozevich, C., and Marshall, T. (1983) Behavioural and Physiological Effects of Ethanol in High-risk and Control Children: A Pilot Study. *Alcoholism* (New York) Fall, 7 (4): 436–42.

Belinkoff, S. and Hall, O. W. Jr. (1950) Intravenous Alcohol in Labor. *American Journal of Obstetrics and Gynecology* 59: 429.

Berger, P. (1981) *Invitation to Sociology: A Humanistic Perspective*. Harmondsworth: Pelican Books.

Berger, P. L. and Kellner, H. (1982) *Sociology Reinterpreted: An Essay on Vocation*. Harmondsworth: Pelican Books.

Berkowitz, G. S. (1981) An Epidemiologic Study of Preterm Delivery. *American Journal of Epidemiology* 113 (1): 81–92.

Berkowitz, G. S., Holford, T. R., and Berkowitz, R. L. (1982) Effects of Cigarette Smoking, Alcohol, Coffee and Tea Consumption on Preterm Delivery. *Early Human Development* 7 (3): 239–50.

Bernard, J. (1982) *The Female World*. New York: The Free Press.

Berner, L. (1977) The Importance of Direct Intervention. *American Journal of Public Health* 67: 1135–136.

Berridge, V. and Edwards, G. (1981) *Opium and the People*. London: Allen Lane.

Bessey, W. E. (1872) On the Use of Alcoholic Stimulants by Nursing Mothers. *Canadian Medical Record* 1: 195.

Beverage Alcohol Information Council (1979) *Public Education Program on Drinking and Pregnancy*. Washington, DC.

Beyers, N. and Moosa, A. (1978) The Fetal Alcohol Syndrome. *South African Medical Journal* 54: 575.

Bezzola, D. (1902) Statistiche Untersuchungen über die Rolle des Alkohols bei der Entstehung des originaren Schwachsinns (Statistical Studies Regarding the Role of Alcohol in the Condition of Original Pregnancy). In *Bericht über den VIII Internationalen Kongress gegen den Alkoholismus* (Vienna) 109–11.

Bianchine, J. W. and Taylor, B. D. (1974) Noonan Syndrome and FAS. *Lancet* 1: 933.

Bieniarz, J., Burd, L., Motew, M., and Scommeg, N. A. (1971) Inhibition of Uterine Contractivity in Labour. *American Journal of Obstetrics and Gynecology* 3: 874.

Bierich, J. R., Majewski, F., and Michaelis, R. (1975) Fetal Alcohol Syndrome. *Pediatric Resident* 9: 864.

—— (1978) Pranatale Schadegungen durch Alkohol (Prenatal Damages from Alcohol). *Internist* 19: 131.

Binkiewicz, A., Robinson, M. J., and Senior, B. (1978) Pseudo-Cushing Syndrome Caused by Alcohol in Breast Milk. *Journal of Pediatrics* 93: 965.

Black, C. (ed.) (1983) *Married Women's Work*. London: Virago.

Black, J. (1983) Drinking Habits During Pregnancy. *Nursing Times* 31 August: 25–6.

Bleicher, S. J. and Waltman, R. (1970) Ethanol Infusions. *Lancet* 1: 1404.

Blinick, G., Wallach, R. C., Jerez, E., and Ackerman, B. D. (1976) Drug Addiction in Pregnancy and the Neonate. *American Journal of Obstetrics and Gynecology* 125: 135.

Bodendorfer, T. W., Briggs, G. C., and Gunning J. (1979) Obtaining Drug Exposure Histories During Pregnancy. *American Journal of Obstetrics and Gynecology* 135: 490–94.

Bond, N. (1978) Fetal Alcohol Syndrome. *Medical Journal of Australia* 65: 164.

Bonn, B. G. (1978) Alcohol and the Fetus. *Maryland State Medical Journal* 27: 21.

Borg, S. and Lasker, J. (1982) *When Pregnancy Fails*. London: Routledge & Kegan Paul.

Borgstedt, A. D. and Rosen, M. G. (1968) Medication During Labor Correlated with Behavior and EEG of the Newborn. *American Journal of Diseases of Childhood* 115: 21.

Boreyru, J. P. (1967) 'La Toxicomanie Alcoolique Parentale et les Répercussions sur la Descendance' ('Prenatal Alcohol Addication and its Effects on Offspring'). Ph.D. Thesis, University of Nantes, France.

Bosma, W. G. H. (1972) Children of Alcoholics: A Hidden Tragedy. *Maryland State Medical Journal* 21: 34–6.

Bottoms, S. F., Judge, N. E., Kuhnert, P. M., and Sokol, R. J. (1982) Thiocyanate and Drinking in Pregnancy. *Alcoholism: Clinical and Experimental Research* 6 (3): 391–95.

Bourne, G. (1975) *Pregnancy*. London: Pan Books.

Boyd, C. and Sellers, S. L. (1982) *The British Way of Birth*. London: Pan Books.

Bradbeer, R., De Bono, P., and Laurie, P. (1982) *The Computer Book*. London: BBC Publications.

The Brewer's Society (1982) *UK Statistical Handbook*. London: Brewing Publications.

Brown, N. A., Goulding, E. H., and Fabro, S. (1979) Ethanol Embryo Toxicity: Direct Effects on Mammalian Embryos *in Vitro*. *Science* 206: 573.

Brunt, R. and Rowan, C. (eds) (1982) *Feminism, Culture and Politics*. London: Lawrence and Wishart.

Brush, M. (1984) *Understanding Pre-Menstrual Tension*. London: Pan Books.

Brzecka, K., Wachnik, S., and Wiercinski, J. (1977) Narazenie Podu na Etanol w Oparciu o Jego Rosprzestryemaniesiest u Kobiet Ciezarnych (Exposure of the Fetus to Ethanol Estimated on the Basis of the Rate of Alcohol Distribution in a Pregnant Woman). *Problemy Alkoholizma* 24: 5.

Buckalew, L. W. (1978) Effect of Maternal Alcohol Consumption During Nursing on Offspring Activity. *Research Communications in Psychology, Psychiatry and Behavior* 3: 353.

Burke, J. P. and Fenton, M. R. (1978) The Effect of Maternal Ethanol Consumption on Aldehyde Dehydrogenase Activity in Neonates. *Research Communications in Psychology, Psychiatry and Behavior* 3: 169.

Burrows, G. N. and Ferris, T. F. (1975) *Medical Complications During Pregnancy*. Philadelphia, Pa.: W. B. Saunders.

Bursey, R. G. (1978) 'Effect of Maternal Ethanol Consumption during Gestation and Lactation on the Development and Learning Preference of the Offspring.' Ph.D. Thesis, Clemson University: Clemson, South Carolina.

Burton, R. (1906) (originally published in 1621) The Causes of Melancholy in *The Anatomy of Melancholy* Vol 1, Part 1, Section 2. London: William Tegg.

Butler, F. O. (1942) The Defective Delinquent. *American Journal of Mental Deficiency* 47: 7–13.

Butler, P. E. (1981) *Self-Assertion for Women*. San Francisco, Calif.: Harper and Row.

Cadotte, M., Allard, S., and Verdy, M. (1973) Lack of Effect of Ethanol *in Vitro* on Human Chromosomes. *American Genetics* 16: 55.

CAGE Questionnaire. Validation of a New Alcoholism Screening Instrument. *American Journal of Psychiatry* 131: 1121–123.

Cahalan, D., Cisin, I. H., and Crossley, H. M. (1969) *American Drinking Practices: A National Study of Drinking Behavior and Attitudes*. New Jersey: Publications Division, Rutgers Centre of Alcohol Studies.

Cahalan, D. and Treiman, B. (1976) *Drinking Behavior, Attitudes and Problems in San Francisco*. Report Prepared for Bureau of Alcoholism, Department of Public Health, City and County of San Francisco.

Camberwell Council on Alcoholism (eds) (1980) *Women and Alcohol*. London: Tavistock.

Campbell-Jones, S. (1983) *Horizon at the Frontiers of Medicine*. London: BBC Publications.

Carden, J. H. (1977) Alcool, Grossesse et Morbidité Féto-Infantile (Alcohol, Pregnancy and Fetal-Infantile Morbidity). *Revue de l'Alcoolisme* 23: 201.

Caritis, S. N., Edelstone, D. I., and Mueller-Heubach, C. (1979) Pharmacologic Inhibition of Preterm Labor. *American Journal of Obstetrics and Gynecology* 133: 557.

Castro-Gago, M., Roderiguez-Cervilla, J., Ugarte, J., Novo, I., and Pombo, M. (1984) Maternal Alcohol Ingestion and Neural Tube Defects (letter). *Journal of Pediatrics* 104 (5): 796–97.

Caussade, L., Weimann, N., and Blane, H. (1940) Fails Relatifs à l'alcoolisme Infantile (Failures Relating to Infantile Alcoholism). *Pediatrie* 38: 531.

Cavenagh, J. (1983) The Trade Debate. In M. Grant and E. Ritson (eds), *Alcohol: The Prevention Debate*. London: Croom Helm.

Cavender, D. R. and Clegg, M. T. (1978) Dynamics of Correlated Genetic Systems: IV: Multilocus Effects of Ethanol Stress Environments. *Genetics* 90: 629.

Ceni, C. (1904) Influenza Dell' Alcoolismo sul Potere di Procreare e sui Discendenti (The Influence of Alcohol on the Ability to Reproduce and on the Descendants). *Revista Sperimentale di Freniatria E Medicine Legale Delle Alienazioni Mentali Italia* 30: 339.

Chafetz, M. E. (1965) *Liquor: The Servant of Man*. Boston, Mass.: Little, Brown.

Chafetz, M. E., Blane, H. T., and Hill, M. J. (1971) Children of Alcoholics: Observations in a Child Guidance Clinic. *Quarterly Journal Studies on Alcohol* 32: 687–98.

Chapman, E. R. and Williams, P. T. (1951) Intravenous Alcohol as an Obstetrical Analgesia. *American Journal of Obstetrics and Gynecology* 61 (3): 676–79.

Char, F. (1976) Fetal Alcohol Syndrome with Noonan Phenotype. *Birth Defects* 12: 81.

Charlton, J. R. H., Hartley, R. M., Silver, R., and Holland, W. W. (1983) Geographical Variations in Mortality from Conditions Amenable to Medical Intervention in England and Wales. *Lancet* March 26: 691–96.

Chasnoff, I. J., Diggs, G., and Schnoll, S. H. (1981) Fetal Alcohol Effects and Maternal Cough Syrup Abuse. *American Journal of Diseases of Childhood* 135: 1066.

Chasseguet-Smirgel, J. (1981) *Female Sexuality*. London: Virago.

Chernoff, G. F. (1975) A Mouse Model of the Fetal Alcohol Syndrome. *Teratology* 11: 14a.

—— (1977) The Fetal Alcohol Syndrome in Mice: Maternal Variables. *Teratology* 15: 223–29.

—— (1980) Introduction: A Teratologist's View of the Fetal Alcohol

Syndrome. In M. Galanter (ed.) *Currents in Alcoholism vol. 7: Recent Advances in Research and Treatment*. New York: Grune & Stratton.

Chernoff, G. F. and Lyons Jones, K. (1981) Fetal Preventative Medicine: Teratogens and the Unborn Baby. *Pediatric Annals* 10 (6): 16–27.

Chetwynd, S. J. and Pearson, V. (1983) Alcohol Problems among Women Working in the Home: Prevalence and Predictors. *Australia and New Zealand Journal of Psychiatry* 17 (3): 259–64.

Chick, J., Kreitman, N., and Plant, M. A. (1981) Mean Cell Volume and Gamma-Glutamyl-Transpeptidiase as Markers of Drinking in Working Men. *Lancet* 1: 1249–251.

Child, D. (1970) *The Essentials of Factor Analysis*. London: Holt, Rinehart & Winston.

Christiaens, L. (1961) La Descendance des Alcooliques (The Offspring of Alcoholics). *American Pediatrics* 37: 380.

Christiaens, L., Mizon, J. P., and Delmarle, G. (1960) Sur la Descendance des Alcooliques (On the Offspring of Alcoholics). *American Pediatrics* 36: 37.

Christoffel, K. K. and Salafsky, I. (1975) Fetal Alcohol Syndrome in Dizygotic Twins. *Journal of Pediatrics* 86: 963–67.

Ciba Foundation (1984) *Mechanisms of Alcohol Damage in Utero*. Bath: Pitman Press.

Clarren, S. K. (1978) Central Nervous System Malformation in Two Offspring of Alcoholic Women. *Birth Defects* 13: 151.

—— (1979) Neural Tube Defects and Fetal Alcohol Syndrome. *Journal of Pediatrics* 98: 328.

—— (1982) The Diagnosis and Treatment of FAS. *Comprehensive Therapy* 8 (10): 41–6.

Clarren, S. K. and Alvord, E. C. (1976) Leptomeningeal Neuroglial Heterotopias in Infants of Alcoholic Mothers. *Journal of Neuropathological and Experimental Neurology* 35: 372.

Clarren, S. K. and Smith, D. W. (1978) Medical Progress. The Fetal Alcohol Syndrome. *New England Journal of Medicine* 298 (19): 1063–067.

—— (1978) The Fetal Alcohol Syndrome. *Lamp* 35: 4.

Clarren, S. K., Alvord E. C. Jnr, Sumi, S. M., Streissguth, A. P., and Smith, D. W. (1978) Brain Malformations Related to Prenatal Exposure to Ethanol. *Journal of Pediatrics* 92 (1): 64–7.

Clarren, S. K. and Smith, D. W. (1978) The FAS: Reply to Letter to the Editor. *New England Journal of Medicine* 298: 556.

Clarren, S. K. and Bowden, D. M. (1982) FAS: A New Primate Model for Binge Drinking and its Relevance to Human Ethanol Tolerance. *The Journal of Pediatrics* 101 (5): 819–25.

Cobo, E. (1973) Effect of Different Doses of Ethanol on the Milk-Ejecting Reflex in Lactating Women. *American Journal of Obstetrics and Gynecology* 115 (6): 817–21.

Goffey, T. G. (1966) Beer Street; Gin Lane: Some views of 18th Century Drinking. *Quarterly Journal of Studies on Alcohol* **27**: 669-692.

Cole, L. J. and Davis, C. L. (1914) The Effect of Alcohol on the Male Germ Cells, Studied by Means of Double Matings. *Science* **39**: 476-77.

Collins, E. and Turner, G. (1978) Six Children Affected by Maternal Alcoholism. *Medical Journal of Australia* **2**: 606.

Comfort, A. (1984) Alcohol as a Social Drug and Health Hazard. *Lancet* 25 Febuary (1): (8374) 443-44.

Commission of the European Communities (1979) *The Medico-Social Risks of Alcohol Consumption*. Luxembourg: Commission of the European Communities.

Connolly, T. G. and Sluckin, W. (1971) *An Introduction to Statistics for the Social Sciences*: Third Edition. London: Macmillan.

Cook, L. N., Schott, R. J., and Andrews, B. F. (1975) Acute Transplacental Ethanol Intoxication. *American Journal of Diseases of Childhood* **129**: 1075.

Cooper, P. (1978) Alcohol and the Fetus. *Food Cosmetic Toxicology* **16**: 290.

Cooper, S. J. (1978) Poisoned People: Psychotropic Drugs in Pregnancy: Morphological and Psychological Adverse Effects on Offspring. *Journal of Biosocial Science* **10** (3): 321-34.

Coote, A. and Campbell, B. (1982) *Sweet Freedom: The Struggle for Women's Liberation*. London: Pan Books.

Cork, R. M. (1969) *The Forgotten Children*. Toronto: Paperbacks.

Corrigan, G. E. (1976) Fetal Alcohol Syndrome. *Texas Medicine* **72**: 72-4.

Cosper, R. (1969) Interviewer Bias in a Study of Drinking Practices. *Quarterly Journal Studies on Alcohol* **30**: 152-57.

Coyle, I. R., Wayner, M. J., and Singer, G. (1976) Behavioral Teratogenesis: A Critical Evaluation. *Pharmacology, Biochemistry and Behavior* **4**: 191.

Crawford, A., Kreitman, N., Latcham, R., and Plant, M. A. (1984) Regional Variations in British Alcohol Morbidity Rates: A Myth Uncovered? II. Population Surveys. *British Medical Journal* **289**: 1343-45.

Crocker, A. C. (1982) Current Strategies in Prevention of Mental Retardation. *Paediatric Annals* **11**: 450-57.

Crothers, T. D. (1887) Inebriety Traced to the Intoxication of Parents at the Time of Conception. *Medical and Surgical Report* **56**: 549.

—— (1909) Heredity in the Causation of Inebriety. *British Medical Journal* **2**: 659-61.

Cruz-Coke, R. and Varela, A. (1966) Inheritance of Alcoholism: Its Association with Colour Blindness. *Lancet* **2**: 1282-284.

Czeizel, E. (1978) Az Alkoholista nok Terhessegenek Epidemiologiai Vizagalata (Epidemiological Investigation of Pregnancy among Women Alcoholics). *Alkohologia* **9**: 12.

Dalton, K. (1982) *Once a Month*. England: Fontana.

Daly, M. (1979) *Gyn/Ecology*. London: The Women's Press.

Danforth, C. H. (1919) Evidence that Germ Cells are Subject to Selection on the Bases of their Genetic Patient Abilities. *Journal Experimental Zoology* 28: 385.

Darby, B. L., Streissguth, A. P., and Smith, D. W. (1981) A Preliminary Follow up of 8 Children Diagnosed Fetal Alcohol Syndrome in Infancy. *Neurobehavioral Toxicology and Teratology* 3 (2): 157–59.

Davenport, C. B. (1932) Effects of Alcohol on Animal Offspring. In H. Emerson (ed.) *Alcohol and Man*. New York: Macmillan Inc.

Davidson, S., Alden, L., and Davidson, P. (1981) Changes in Alcohol Consumption after Childbirth. *Journal of Advanced Nursing* 6: 195–98.

Davies, B. L. and Boniface, W. J. (1979) Prenatal Testing for Birth Defects and Nursing Practice. *Journal of Advanced Nursing* 4: 485–91.

Davies, J. B. and Stacey, B. (1972) Teenagers and Alcohol, London: HMSO.

Davies, P. J. M., Partridge, J. W., and Storrs, C. N. (1982) Alcohol Consumption in Pregnancy. How Much is Safe? *Archives of Diseases in Childhood* 57: 940–43.

Davies, P. T. (1982) The Pattern of Problems. In M. A. Plant (ed.) *Drinking and Problem Drinking*. London: Junction.

Davies, P. T. and Walsh, D. (1983) *Alcohol Problems and Alcohol Control in Europe*. London: Croom Helm.

Davis, A. (1981) *Let's Have Healthy Children*. London: Allen & Unwin.

Davis, K. (1977) Alcohol Linked to Birth Defects. *National Council on Alcoholism* Reports 1: 1.

De Beauvoir, S. (1982) *The Woman Destroyed*. Glasgow: William Collins.

Debeukelaer, M. M. and Randall, C. L. (1977) The Fetal Alcohol Syndrome. *Journal South Carolina Medical Association* 73: 407.

Debeukelaer, M. M., Randall, C. L., and Stroud, D. R. (1977) Renal Anomalies in the FAS. *Journal of Pediatrics* 91: 759.

De Chateau, P. (1977) Ett Fal av Etylfetapati (On the Fetal Alcohol Syndrome). *Lakartidningen* 72: 1933.

Dehaene, P. H., Crepin, G., Walbaum, R., Titran, M., Samaille-Villette, C. H., and Samaille, P. (1977) Le Descendance des Mères Alcooliques Chroniques. A Propos de 16 Cas D'Alcoolisme Foetal (Offspring of Chronic Alcoholic Mothers: A Report of 16 Cases of Fetal Alcoholism). *Revue Française De Gynécologie et d'Obstétrique* 72: 492.

Dehaene, P., Samaille-Villette, C., Samaille, P., Crespin G., Walbaum R., Deroubaix, P., Blanc-Garin, A. P. (1977) Le Syndrome D'Alcoolisme Foetal Dans le Nord de la France (The FAS in the North of France). *Revue de l'Alcoolisme* 23: 145–58.

Dehaene, P. H, Crepin, G., Delahousse, G., Querleu, Walbaum, R., Titran, M., and Samaille-Villette, C. (1981) Aspects Epidémiologiques Du Syndrome D'Alcoolisme Foetal. *La Nouvelle Press Médicale* 10 (32): 2639–643.

Dehaene, P., Titran, M., Samaille-Villette, C., Samaille, P., Crespin, G., Delahousse, G., Walbaum, R., Fasquelle, P. (1977) Fréquence du Syndrome D'Alcoolisme Foetal (Frequency of the FAS). *La Nouvelle Presse Médicale* (Paris) **20**: 1763.

Deibel, P. (1980) Effects of Cigarette Smoking on Maternal Nutrition and the Fetus. *Journal of Obstetrics and Gynecological Nursing* 9 (6): 333–36.

Delamont, S. (1980) *The Sociology of Women*. London: Allen & Unwin.

Dendy, M. (1910) Letter on the Notes made by Dr Ashby concerning Manchester Children and Furnished to Elderton and Pearson. *British Medical Journal* 1 (50): 348.

Denmark, L. D. (1954) Smoking and Drinking During Pregnancy. *Journal of the American Medical Association* **154**: 186.

Department of Health and Social Security (1981) *Drinking Sensibly*. London: HMSO.

—— (1983) *Prevention and Health: Everybody's Business*. London: HMSO.

Department of Health, Education and Welfare (1977) The Fetal Alcohol Syndrome. *Food and Drug Administration Drug Bulletin* 18.

Department of Treasury, Bureau of Alcohol, Tobacco and Firearms (1979) *FAS: Public Awareness Campaign*. Washington, DC: US Government Printing Office.

Desmond, M. M., Rudolph, A. J., Hill, R. M., Claghorn, J. I., Greesen, P. R., and Burgdorff, I. (1969) *Behavioral Alterations in Infants Born to Mothers on Psychoactive Drugs during Pregnancy*. Austin: University of Texas Press.

Desmond, M. M. and Wilson, G. S. (1975) Neonatal Abstinence Syndrome: Recognition and Diagnosis. *Addictive Diseases* **2**: 113.

Detering, N., Collins, R., Ozand, P. T., and Karahasan, A. M. (1979) The Effects of Ethanol (E) on Developing Catecholamine Neurons. *Alcoholism: Clinical and Experimental Research* **3**: 276.

Detorek, D. (1972) Chromosomal Irregularities in Alcoholics. *Annals New York Academy of Science* **197**: 90.

Dickens, G. and Trethowan, W. H. (1971) Cravings and Aversions During Pregnancy. *Journal of Psychosomatic Research* **15**: 259.

Dickson, A. (1982) *A Woman in Your Own Right*. London: Quartet Books.

Dight, S. (1976) *Scottish Drinking Habits*. London: HMSO.

Dilts, P. V. Jnr (1970a) Placental Transfer of Ethanol. *American Journal of Obstetrics and Gynecology* **107**: 1195.

—— (1970b) Effects of Ethanol on Maternal and Fetal Acid-Base Balance. *American Journal of Obstetrics and Gynecology* **107**: 1018.

—— (1970c) Effect of Ethanol on External and Fetal Umbilical Haemodynamics and Oxygen Transfer. *American Journal of Obstetrics and Gynecology* **106**: 221.

Dobie, J. and Bill, P. (1977) Fetal Alcohol Syndrome. *Addictions* (Toronto) **24**: 5–15.

Dobbing, J. and Sands, J. (1979) Comparative Aspects of Growth and

Sport. *Early Human Development* 3: 79–83.

Dowdell, P. M. (1981) Alcohol and Pregnancy – A Review of the Literature 1968–80. *Nursing Times* 21 October: 1825–831.

Dowling, C. (1981) *The Cinderella Complex.* London: Fontana.

Driscoll, G. Z. and Barr, H. L. (1972) *Comparative Study of Drug Dependent and Alcoholic Women.* Selected Papers of the 23rd Annual Meeting of the Alcohol and Drug Problems Association of North America.

Duffy, J. (1982) (Personal Communication).

Dumont, M. (1977) Ethanol Perfusions During Threatened Premature Labor – Special Study of Oxytocinase Activity. *Journal de Gynécologique, Obstétrique et Biologique de la Reproduction* (Paris) 6: 107–16.

Dumont, N. (1977) Hypotrophie Foetale et Intoxications Maternelles Chroniques (Fetal Hypotrophy and Chronic Maternal Intoxication). *Revue Française De Gynécologie et D'Obstétrique* 72: 797.

Dunham, R. G. (1983) Rethinking the Measurement of Drinking Patterns. *Journal of Studies in Alcohol* 44 (3): 485–93.

Dunn, P. M. (1979) Metronidiazole and the FAS. *Lancet* 2: 134.

Dupuis, C., Dehaene, P., Deroubaix-Tella, P., Blanc-Garin, A. P., Rey, C., and Carpentier-Couralt, C. (1978) Les Cardiopathies des Enfants nés de Mère Alcoolique (The Heart Diseases of Children born to Alcoholic Mothers). *Archives Des Maladies du Coeur et des Vaisseaux* 71; 5; 656–72.

Durham, F. M. and Woods, N. M. (1932) *Alcohol and Inheritance: An Experimental Study.* Medical Research Council, Special Report Series, No. 168. London: HMSO.

Eaves, L., Nuttall, J., Klonoff, H., and Dunn, H. (1970) Developmental and Psychological Test Scores in Children of Low Birth Weight. *Pediatrics* 49: 9.

Eckardt, M. J., Harford, T. C., Kaelber, C. T., Parker, E. S., Rosenthal, L. S., Ryback, R. S., Salmoiraghi, G. C., Vanderveen, E., and Warren, K. R. (1981) Health Hazards Associated with Alcohol Consumption. *Journal of the American Medical Association* 246 (6): 648–65.

Edelson, E. (1977) With Child? Don't Drink, Group Says. *National Council on Alcoholism Reports* June 19: 1.

Editorial (1976) Fetal Alcohol Syndrome. *British Medical Journal* 2: 1404.

Editorial (1976) Fetal Alcohol Syndrome. *Lancet* 2: 1335.

Editorial (1977) Pregnancy in the Heavy Drinker. *Lancet* 2: 647.

Editorial (1977) The Fetal Alcohol Syndrome. *Alcoholism: Clinical and Experimental Research* 1: 191.

Editorial (1978) Warnings Needed Now: The Fetal Alcohol Syndrome. *All Faith's World Alcohol Project Journal* 1: 47.

Editorial (1979) Born to Drink. *Lancet* 1: 24.

Editorial (1980) Low Birth Weight, Drink, Smoking and Diet. *Public Health* 97 (6): 307–8.

Edwards, G. (1983) Alcohol and Advice to Pregnant Women. *British Medical Journal* **286**: 247–48.

Edwards, G., Arif, A., and Jaffe, J. (eds) (1983) *Drug Use and Misuse: Cultural Perspectives.* Beckenham: Croom Helm.

Edwards, J. (1847) *A Temperance Manual.* New York: American Tract Society.

Ehrenreich, B. and English, D. (1979) *For Her Own Good: 150 Years of the Experts' Advice to Women.* London: Pluto Press.

Ehrlich, W. (1910) 'La Postérité des Alcooliques' ('The Offspring of Alcoholics'). Thesis, Lausanne.

Eichenbaum L. and Orbach, S. (1982) *Outside In Inside Out.* Harmondsworth: Pelican Books.

—— (1983) *What Do Women Want?* London: Michael Joseph.

Elbourne, D. (1981) *Is the Baby All Right?* London: Junction Books.

Elderton, E. and Pearson, K. (1910) *A First Study of the Influence of Parental Alcoholism on the Physique and Ability of the Offspring* (Eugenics Laboratory Memoir). London: Cambridge University Press.

El-Guebaly, N. and Offord, D. R. (1977) The Offspring of Alcoholics: A Critical Review. *American Journal of Psychiatry* **134**: 357–65.

—— (1979) On Being the Offspring of an Alcoholic: An Update. *Alcoholism: Clinical and Experimental Research* **3**: 148.

Ellis, J. and Krisiak, M. (1975) Effect of Alcohol Administration During Pregnancy on Social Behavior of Offspring in Mice. *Activitas Nervosa Superior* **17**: 281–82.

Ellis, F. W. and Pick, J. R. (1980) An Animal Model of the Fetal Alcohol Syndrome in Beagles. *Alcoholism: Clinical and Experimental Research* **4**: 123–34.

Ellis, F. W., Pick, J. R., and Sawyer, M. (1977) 'Ethanol Dose-Response Relationships in a Beagle Model of the Fetal Alcohol Syndrome.' Paper Presented at the FAS Workshop, San Diego, California.

English, D. and Bower, C. (1983) Alcohol Consumption, Pregnancy, and Low Birthweight (letter). *Lancet* **1** (8333): 1111.

Epstein, C. F. (1970) *Woman's Place.* London: University of California Press.

Erb, L. and Andresen, B. D. (1978) The Fetal Alcohol Syndrome. *Clinical Pediatrics* **17** (8): 644–49.

Eskes, T. T. (1979) Het Foetale Alcohol Syndrom (The FAS). *Ned Tizdschr Geneeskd* **123**: 1276.

Evans, M. (1982) *The Woman Question.* England: Fontana.

Ewing, J. A. (1968) Alcohol, Sex and Marriage. *Medical Aspects of Human Sexuality* **4**: 43.

Faust, B. (1982) *Women, Sex and Pornography.* Harmondsworth: Pelican Books.

Feldman, B. (1927) Alcohol in Ancient Jewish Literature. *British Journal of Inebriety* **24**: 121–24.

Feldman, S. (1978) *Choices in Childbirth.* New York: Grosset & Dunlop.

Ferguson, M. (1983) *Forever Feminine.* London: Heinemann.

Feroze, R. M. (1983) Alcohol and Pregnancy. *Journal of the Royal College of Obstetrics and Gynaecology.*

Ferrier, P. E. (1979) Fetal Alcohol Syndrome. *Helvetica Paediatric Acta* 34: 105.

―― (1979) Le Syndrome de l'Alcoolisme Foetal (The FAS). *Bulletin Der Schweizerischen Akademie Der Medizinischen Wissenschaften* 35: 145.

Ferrier, P. E., Nicod, I., and Ferrier, S. (1973) Fetal Alcohol Syndrome. *Lancet* 2: 1496.

Fetchko, A. M., Weber, J. E., Carroll, J. H., and Thomas, G. J. (1951) Intravenous Alcohol Used for Pre-Induction Analgesia in Obstetrics. *American Journal of Obstetrics and Gynecology* 62: 662.

Fielding, S. and Yankauer, A. (1978) The Pregnant Drinker. *American Journal of Public Health* 68: 836.

Figa-Talamanca, I. and Modolo, M. A. (1977) A Study of Behavioral Aspects of Infant Mortality in an Italian Community. *International Journal of Health Education* 20: 248.

Figuerido, C. A. (1947) Los Ilamados Males Germinales y los Descendientes de Toxicomones (So-called Germ Damage and the Offspring of Addicts). *Revisita De Sanidad E Higiene Publica* 21: 1215.

Finnegan, L. P., Kron, R. E., Connaughton, J. F., and Emich, J. P. (1975a) A Scoring System for Evaluation and Treatment of the Neonatal Abstinence Syndrome: A New Clinical and Research Tool. In P. L. Morselli, S. Garattini, and F. Serem (eds) *Basic and Therapeutic Aspects of Perinatal Pharmacology.* New York: Raven Press.

―― (1975b) Neonatal Abstinence Syndrome: Assessment and Management. *Addictive Diseases* 2: 141.

―― (1975c) Assessment and Treatment of Abstinence in the Infant of the Drug-Dependent Mother. *International Journal Clinical Pharmacology and Biopharmacology* 12: 19.

Fiocchi, A., Colombini, A., and Codara, L. (1978) La Embriopatia Alcoolica: Rassegna Della Letteratura e Contributo Personale (Alcohol Embryopathy: A Literature Review and Personal Contribution). *Minerva Pediatrica* (Torino) 30: 19–28.

Fischhoff, B., Lichtenstein, S., Slovic, P., Derby, S. L., and Keeney, R. L. (1983) *Acceptable Risk.* Cambridge: Cambridge University Press.

Fisher, S. E., Atkinson, M., Burnap, J. K., Jacobson, S., Sehgal, P. K., Scott, W., and Van Thiel, D. H. (1982) Ethanol-Associated Selective Malnutrition: A Contributing Factor in the Fetal Alcohol Syndrome. *Alcoholism: Clinical and Experimental Research* 6 (2): 197–201.

Fitze, F., Spahr, A., and Pescia, G. (1978) Familienstudie zum Problem des Embryofotalen Alkoholsyndroms (FAS: Follow-Up of a Family). *Schweizer, Rundschau (Praxis)* 67: 1338.

Flynn, A., Miller, S. I., Martier, S. S., Golden, N. L., Sokol, R. J., and

Delvillano, B. C. (1981) Zinc Status of Pregnant Alcoholic Women. A Determinant of Fetal Outcome. *Lancet* 14: 572–74.

Forel, A. (1893) The Effect of Alcoholic Intoxication upon the Human Brain and its Relation to the Theories of Heredity and Evolution. *Quarterly Journal of Inebriety* 12: 203.

Foster, E. (1781) *The Principles and Practices of Midwifery*. London: R. Baldwin.

Fox, H. E., Steinbrecher, M., Pessel, D., Inglis, J., Medvid, L., and Angel, E. (1978) Maternal Ethanol Ingestion and the Occurrence of Human Fetal Breathing Movements. *American Journal of Obstetrics and Gynecology*. 132 (4): 354–58.

Frank, L. M. and Rosman, N. P. (1978) Studies on Growth, Learning and Morphogenesis in Experimental FAS. *American Neurology* 4: 195.

Fransella, F. and Frost, K. (1977) *On Being a Woman*. London: Tavistock.

Frets, G. P. (1931) *Alcohol and the Other Germ Poisons*. The Hague: Nijhoff.

Fried, P. A., Innes, K. S., and Barnes, M. V. (1984) Soft Drug Use Prior to and During Pregnancy: A Comparison of Samples over a 4-year Period. *Drug Alcohol Dependence* 13 (2): 161–76.

Fried, R. I. and Ravin, J. G. (1978) Fetal Alcohol Syndrome. *Journal of Pediatric Ophthalmology* 15: 394.

Friedan, B. (1981) *The Second Stage*. London: Abacus.

—— (1982) *The Feminine Mystique*. Harmondsworth: Pelican Books.

Friedman, J. M. (1982) Can Maternal Alcohol Ingestion Cause Neural Tube Defects? *The Journal of Pediatrics* 101 (2): 232–34.

Fryns, J. P., Deroover, J., Parloir, C., Goffaux, P., Lebas, E., and Van Der Berghe, H. (1977) The Foetal Alcohol Syndrome. *Acta Paediatrica Belgique* 30: 117–21.

Fuchs, F. (1976) Treatment of Imminent Premature Labour (Letter). *Acta Obstetrica Gynecologia Scandinavica* 55: 379.

Fuchs, F. and Wagner, G. (1963) Effects of Alcohol on Release of Oxytocin. *Nature* 198: 92.

Fuchs, F., Fuchs, A. R., Poblete, V. F., and Risk, A. (1967) Effects of Alcohol on Threatened Premature Labour. *American Journal of Obstetrics and Gynaecology* 99 (5): 627–37.

Furey, E. (1982) The Effects of Alcohol on the Fetus. *Exceptional Children* 49 (1): 30–4.

Furnas, J. C. (1965) *The Life and Times of the Late Demon Rum*. London: W. H. Allen.

Fuster, J. S., Guell, S., Cahuana, A. B., and Garciatornel, S. (1979) Neural Tube Defects with FAS. *Journal of Pediatrics* 95: 328.

Gabrielli, W. F. Jnr. and Mednick, S. A. (1983) Intellectual Performance in Children of Alcoholics. *Journal of Nervous and Mental Disorders* 171 (7): 444–47.

Gairdner, D. and Pearson, J. (1971) *Growth and Development Chart*. Hertford: Castlemead Publications.

Gal, P. and Sharpless, M. K. (1984) Fetal Drug Exposure-Behavioral Teratogenesis. *Drug Intelligence and Clinical Pharmacology* March: 18: 3: 186–201.

Gallop, J. (1982) *Feminism and Psychoanalysis*. London: Macmillan.

Galton, F. (1889) *Natural Inheritance*. London: Macmillan.

Game, A. and Pringle, R. (1983) *Gender at Work*. London: Allen & Unwin.

Gardner, R. J. M. and Clarkson, J. E. (1981) A Malformed Child whose Previously Alcoholic Mother Had Taken Disulfiram. *New Zealand Medical Journal* 25 March: 184–86.

Garret, G. R. and Barr, H. M. (1974) Comparison of Self-Rating and Quantity-Frequency Measures of Drinking. *Quarterly Journal Studies on Alcohol* 35: 1293–306.

Garrido-Lestache, J. (1977) La Madre et Alcohol y la Descendencia (The Mother, Alcohol and Offspring). *Anales De La Real Academia Nacional de Medicina* 94: 495.

Gartner, U. and Ryden, G. (1972) The Elimination of Alcohol in the Premature Infant. *Acta Paediatrica Scandinavica* 61: 720–21.

George, M. D. (1965) (originally published 1925) *London Life in the Eighteenth Century*. New York: Capricorn.

Gersh, E. S. and Gersh, I. (1981) *The Biology of Women*. London: Junction Books.

Gibbins, G. L. D. and Chard, T. (1976) Observations on Maternal Oxytocin Release during Labour and the Effect of Intravenous Alcohol Administration. *American Journal of Obstetrics and Gynecology* 124: 243.

Gibbins, R., Israel, Y., Kalant, H., Popham, R. E., Schmidt, W., and Smart, R. G. (1974) *Research Advances in Alcohol and Drug Problems: Vol. One*. New York: John Wiley.

Gibbens, T. C. N. and Walker, A. (1956) *Cruel Parents*. London: Institute for the Study and Treatment of Delinquency.

Gibson, G. T., Baghurst, P. A., and Colley, D. P. (1983) Maternal Alcohol Tobacco and Cannabis Consumption and the Outcome of Pregnancy. *Australia and New Zealand Journal of Obstetrics and Gynaecology* 23: 15–19.

Gilder, S. S. B. (1974) Alcohol, Tobacco and Pregnancy. *Canadian Medical Association Journal* 110: 903.

Gilford, H. (1912) Alcoholism and Problems of Growth and Development. *British Journal of Inebriety* 9: 173.

Gillette, J. R., Menard, R. H., and Stripp, B. (1973) Active Products of Fetal Drug Metabolism. *Clinical Pharmacology and Therapeutics* 14: 680.

Ginsberg, J. (1971) Placental Drug Transfer. *Annual Review of Pharmacology and Toxicology* 11: 387.

Gloor, P. A. (1952) Alcoolisme et Sélection (Alcoholism and Selection). *Schweiz Archiv fur Neurologie, Neurochirurgie und Psychiatrie* 70: 445.

Goetzman, B. W., Kagan, J., and Blankenship, W. J. (1975) Expansion of

136 Women, Drinking, and Pregnancy

the Fetal Alcohol Syndrome. *Clinical Research* **23**: 100.

Gold, S. and Sherry, L. (1984) Hyperactivity, Learning Disabilities and Alcohol. *Journal of Learning Disabilities.* 17 January (1) 3–6.

Goldberg, A. (1984) (Personal Communication).

Golden, N. L., Sokol, R. J., Kuhnert, B. R., and Bottoms, S. F. (1982) Maternal Alcohol Use and Infant Development. *Pediatrics* **70** (6): 931–34.

Goldstein, G. and Arulanantham, K. (1978) Neural Tube Defect and Renal Anomalies in a Child with FAS. *Journal of Pediatrics* **93**: 636.

Gomel, V. and Carpenter, C. W. (1973) Induction of Mid-Trimester Abortion with Intra-Uterine Alcohol. *Obstetrics and Gynaecology* 41 (3): 455–58.

Goodwin, D. W., Schulsinger, F., Hermansen, L., Guze, S. B., and Winokur, G. (1973) Alcohol Problems in Adoptees Raised Apart from Alcoholic Biological Parents. *Archives of General Psychiatry* **28**: 238–43.

—— (1975) Alcoholism and the Hyperactive Child Syndrome. *Journal of Nervous and Mental Diseases* **160**: 349–53.

Goodwin, D. W. (1983) The Genetics of Alcoholism. *Hospital Community Psychiatry,* 34: 11: 1031–34.

Gordis, E. and Kreek, M. J. (1977) Alcoholism and Drug Addiction in Pregnancy. *Current Problems in Obstetrics and Gynecology* **I**: 1–48. Chicago, Ill.: Year Book Medical Publishers.

Gordon, A. (1911) Parental Alcoholism as a Factor in the Mental Deficiency of Children: A Statistical Study of 117 Families. *Journal of Inebriety* **33**: 90–9.

—— (1913) Parental Alcoholism as a Factor in the Mental Deficiency of Children: Follow-up. *Journal of Inebriety* **35**: 58–65.

—— (1916) The Influence of Alcohol on the Progenitor. *International Medical Journal* **23**: 431.

Gordon, G. G., Altman, K., Southren, A. L., Rubin, E., and Lieber, C. S. (1976) Effect of Alcohol (Ethanol) Administration on Sex Hormone Metabolism in Normal Men. *New England Journal of Medicine* **295**: 793.

Gordon, G. G., Southren, A. L., and Lieber, C. S. (1978) The Effects of Alcoholic Liver Disease and Alcohol Ingestion on Sex Hormone Levels. *Alcoholism: Clinical and Experimental Research* **2**: 259.

Goujard, J., Kaminski, M., Rumeau-Rouquette, C. and Schwartz, D. (1978) Maternal Smoking, Alcohol Consumption and Abruptio Placentae. *American Journal of Obstetrics and Gynecology* **130**: 738.

Graff, G. (1971) Failure to Prevent Premature Labour with Ethanol. *American Journal of Obstetrics and Gynecology* **110**: 878.

Graham-Clay, S. (1983) FAS: A Review of the Current Human Research. *Canada's Mental Health* June: 2–5.

Grant, E. C. G. (1981) The Harmful Effects of Common Social Habits Especially Smoking and Using Oral Contraceptive Steroids on Pregnancy. *International Journal of Environmental Studies* **17**: 57–66.

Grant, M. (1982a) The Trade Debate. In M. Grant and E. B. Ritson, *Alcohol: The Prevention Debate*. London: Croom Helm.

—— (1982b) Prevention. In M. A. Plant (ed) *Drinking and Problem Drinking*. London: Croom Helm.

Grant, M., Plant, M. A., and Williams, A. (eds) (1983) *Economics and Alcohol*. Beckenham: Croom Helm.

Grant, M. and Ritson, E. B. (eds) (1983) *Alcohol: The Prevention Debate*. London: Croom Helm.

Green, H. G. (1974) Infants of Alcoholic Mothers. *American Journal of Obstetrics and Gynecology* 118: 713–16.

Greenblatt, M. and Schuckit, M. (eds) (1976) *Alcoholism Problems in Women and Children*. New York: Grune & Stratton.

Greenhouse, B. S., Hook, R. and Hehre, F. W. (1969) Aspiration Pneumonia Following Intravenous Administration of Alcohol During Labor. *Journal of the American Medical Association* 210: 168.

Greizerstein, H. B., Abel, E. L., and Siemens, A. J. (1979) Lactation and Ethanol Disappearance in the Rat. *Pharmacologist* 21: 188. (Abstract 233.)

Grenier, L. (1881) 'Contribution à l'Etude, de la Descendance des Alcooliques' ('Contribution to the Study of the Offspring of the Alcoholic'). Thesis, Paris.

Gurling, H. M. (1984) Genetic Epidemiology in Medicine – Recent Twin Research (editorial). *British Medical Journal* (Clinical-Research) 288 (6410): 3–5.

Gusella, J. L. and Fried, P. A. (1984) Effects of Maternal Social Drinking and Smoking on Offspring at 13 Months. *Neurobehavioral-Toxicology and Teratology* 6 (1): 13–17.

Gutzke, D. W. (1984) 'The Cry of the Children': The Edwardian Medical Campaign against Maternal Drinking. *British Journal of Addiction* 79 (1): 71–84.

Habbick, B. F., Zaleski, W., Casey, R., and Murphy, F. (1979) Liver Abnormalities in Three Patients with Fetal Alcohol Syndrome. *Lancet* March: 580–81.

Haberman, P. W. (1966) Childhood Symptoms in Children of Alcoholics and Comparison Group Parents. *Journal of Marriage and the Family* 28: 152–54.

Haddon, J. (1876) On Intemperance in Women, with Special Reference to its Effects on the Reproductive System. *British Medical Journal* 1: 748–50.

Haggard, H. W. and Jellinek, E. M. (1942) *Alcohol Explored*. New York: Doubleday.

Hall, B. D. and Orenstein, W. A. (1974) Noonan's Phenotype in an Offspring of an Alcoholic Mother. *Lancet* 1: 680.

Hall, R. (ed.) (1981) *Dear Dr Stopes*. Harmondsworth: Penguin Books.

Halliday, H. L., McClure, G., and Reid, M.Mc. (1983) Alcohol and the Fetus. *Lancet* 30 April: 984.

138   *Women, Drinking, and Pregnancy*

Halliday, H. L., Reid, M.Mc., and McClure, G. (1982) Results of Heavy
Drinking in Pregnancy. *British Journal of Obstetrics and Gynaecology*
89: 892–95.

Halmi, K. A. and Loney, J. (1973) Familial Alcoholism in Anorexia
Nervosa. *British Journal of Psychiatry* 123: 53–4.

Hann, J. (1982) *The Perfect Baby?* London: Weidenfeld & Nicolson.

Hanson, J. W. (1977) Alcohol and the Fetus. *British Journal of Hospital
Medicine* August: 126–30.

Hanson, J. W., Jones, K. L., and Smith, D. W. (1976) Fetal Alcohol Syndrome, Experience with 41 Patients. *Journal of the American Medical
Association* 235: 1458–60.

Hanson, J. W., Jones, K. L., and Smith, D. W. (1976) Fetal Alcohol
Syndrome. *Journal of the American Medical Association* 236: 1114.

Hanson, J. W., Streissguth, A. P., and Smith, D. W. (1978) The Effects of
Moderate Alcohol Consumption during Pregnancy on Fetal Growth and
Morphogenesis. *Journal of Pediatrics* 92; 457–60.

Harding, M. E. (1982) *Woman's Mysteries: Ancient and Modern*. London:
Rider.

Harlap, S., Shiono, P. H., and Ramcharan, S. (1979) Alcohol and Spontaneous Abortions. *American Journal of Epidemiology* 110: 372.
(Abstract.)

Harlap, S. and Shiona, P. H. (1980) Alcohol, Smoking and the Incidence of
Spontaneous Abortions in the First and Second Trimester. *Lancet* 2:
173–76.

Harpwood, D. (1982) *Tea and Tranquillisers*. London: Virago.

Harries, J. M. and Hughes, T. F. (1958) Enumeration of the 'Cravings' of
Some Pregnant Women. *British Medical Journal* 2: 35.

Harris, P. (ed.) (1977) *The Rhythm of the Glass*. Edinburgh: Paul Harris.

Harris, R. A. and Case, J. (1978) Maternal Consumption of Ethanol
Barbital or Chlordiazepoxide: Effects on Behavior of the Offspring.
Neurosciences Abstract 4: 493.

—— (1979) Effect of Maternal Consumption of Ethanol, Barbital or
Chlordiazepoxide on the Behavior of Offspring. *Behavioral and Neural
Biology* 26: 234.

Harrison, M. (1977) *Fire From Heaven*. London: Pan Books.

Hartwig, H., Rohloff, P., Huller, H., and Amon, I. (1982) Drugs in Pregnancy – A Prospective Study. *Biological Research in Pregnancy* 3 (2):
51–5.

Haskey, J. C., Balarajan, R., and Donnan, S. P. B. (1983) Regional Variations in Alcohol Related Problems within the United Kingdom. *Community Medicine* 5: 208–19.

Havlicek, V. and Childiaeva, R. (1976) EEG Component of Fetal Alcohol
Syndrome. *Lancet* 2: 477.

Havlicek, V., Chiladiaeva, R., and Chernick, W. (1977) EEG Frequency
Spectrum Characteristics of Sleep Rates in Infants of Alcoholic Mothers.
Neuropaediatrics 8: 360.

Hayden, M. R. and Nelson, M. M. (1978) The Fetal Alcohol Syndrome. *South African Medical Journal* 54: 571.

Heather, N. and Robertson, I. (1981) *Controlled Drinking*. London: Methuen.

HEC (1983) *That's the Limit*. London: Health Education Council for England and Wales.

Heine, M. W. (1981) Alcoholism and Reproduction. *Progress in Biochemical Pharmacology* 18: 75–82.

Hemminki, E. and Starfield, B. (1978) Prevention and Treatment of Premature Labour by Drugs: Review of Controlled Clinical Trials. *British Journal of Obstetrics and Gynaecology* 85: 411.

Herman, C. S., Kirchner, G. L., Streissguth, A. P., and Little, R. E. (1980) Vigilance Paradigm for Preschool Children Used to Relate Vigilance Behavior to IQ and Prenatal Exposure to Alcohol. *Perceptual and Motor Skills* 50: 863–67.

Hermier, M., Leclercq, F., Duc, H., David, L., and François, R. (1976) Le Nanisme Intra-Utérin avec Débilité Mentale et Malformations dans le Cadre de L'Embryo-Foetopathie Alcoolique à Propos de Quatre Cas (Intrauterine Growth Deficiency with Mental Retardation and Malformations in Alcoholic Embry-Fetopathy – 4 Cases). *Pédiatrie* 31: 749.

Heuyer, O., Mises, R., and Dereux, J. F. (1957) Le Descendance des Alcooliques (The Offspring of Alcoholics). *Nouvelle Presse Médicale* 29: 657.

Hill, R. M., Craig, J. P., Chaney, M. D., Tennyson, L. M., and McCulley, L. B. (1977) Utilisation of Over-The-Counter Drugs during Pregnancy. *Clinical Obstetrics and Gynecology* 20 (2): 381–94.

Himwich, W. A., Hall, J. S., and MacArthur, W. F. (1977) Maternal Alcohol and Neonatal Health. *Biological Psychiatry* 12 (4): 495–505.

Hinckers, H. J. (1978) The Influences of Alcohol on the Fetus. *Journal of Perinatal Medicine* 6 (1): 3–14.

Hingson, R. (1982) Personal communication.

Hingson, R. (1983) FAS-Like Symptoms Seen in Pot-Smokers Newborn? *The Journal* 1 January: 2.

Hingson, R., Alpert, J. J., Day, N., Dooling, E., Kayne, H., Morelock, S., Oppenheimer, E., and Zuckermann, B. (1982) 'Effects of Maternal Drinking and Marijuana Use on Fetal Growth and Development.' Paper Presented at ICAA Alcohol Epidemiology Section Symposium, Helsinki, June/July.

Hingson, R., Alpert, J. J., Day, N., Dooling, E., Kayne, H., Morelock, S., Oppenheimer, E., and Zuckermann, B. (1982) Effects of Maternal Drinking and Marijuana Use on Fetal Growth and Development. *Pediatrics* 70 (4): 539–46.

Hingson, R., Gould, J. B., Morelock, S., Kayne, H., Heeren, T., Alpert, J. J., Zuckerman, B., and Day, N. (1982) Maternal Cigarette Smoking,

Psychoactive Substance Use and Infant Apgar Scores. (Personal communication)

HMSO (1979) *Nurse, Midwives and Health Visitors Act 1979*. London: HMSO.

Ho, B. T., Fritchie, E., Idänpään-Heikkilä, J. E., and McIsaac, W. M. (1972) Placental Transfer and Tissue Distribution of Ethanol-l-14c. *Quarterly Journal Studies on Alcohol* **33**: 485.

Hodge, C. F. (1903) The Influence of Alcohol on Growth and Development. In W. O. Atwater *et al.* (eds) *Physiological Aspects of the Liquor Problems*. Vol. 1. Boston, Mass: Houghton Mifflin.

Hoennicke, A. (1907) Uber Experimentale Erzengte Missbildungen (On Experimentally Created Defects). *Munchener Medizinische Wochenschrif* **2** (54): 2065.

Hollstedt, C. (1975) Ger Alkohol Forsterskador? (Does Alcohol Injure the Fetus?) *Alkohol Och Narkotika* **69**: 123.

Hollstedt, C., Dahlgren, L., and Rydberg, U. (1983) Outcome of Pregnancy in Women Treated at an Alcohol Clinic. *Acta-Psychiatrica Scandinavica* **67** (4): 236–48.

Hollstedt, C., Olsson, O., and Rydberg, U. (1977) The Effect of Alcohol on the Developing Organism: Genetical, Teratological and Physiological Aspects. *Medical Biology* **55**: 1.

Homan, W. E. (1981) *A Report on the FAS: The Bad Mix*. National Institute Alcohol and Alcohol Abuse Information and Feature Service, 1 April: 385–86.

Hoppe, H. (1910) Procreation During Intoxication. *Journal of Inebriety* **32**: 105–10.

Hornstein, L., Crowe, C., and Grupp, O. R. (1977) Adrenal Carcinoma in Child with History of FAS. *Lancet* **2**: 1292.

Howe, S. G. (1848) *Report Made to the Legislature of Massachusetts upon Idiocy*. Boston, Mass.: Coolidge & Wiley.

Howell, J., Clozel, M., and Aranda, V. A. (1981) Adverse Effects of Caffeine and Theophylline in the Newborn Infant. *Seminars on Perinatology* **5** (4) (October): 359–69.

Hugues, J. N., Perret, G., Adessi, I., Coste, T., and Modigliani, E. (1978) Effects of Chronic Alcoholism on the Pituitary-Gonadal Function of Women During Menopausal Transition and in the Post-Menopausal Period. *Biomedicine Express* **29**: 279–83.

Hutter, B. and Williams, G. (1981) *Controlling Women: The Normal and the Deviant*. London: Croom Helm.

Idänpään-Heikkilä, J. E., Fritchie, G. E., Ho, B. T., and McIsaac, W. M. (1971) Placental Transfer of ¹⁴C-Ethanol. *American Journal of Obstetrics and Gynecology* **110**: 426.

Idänpään-Heikkilä, J., Jouppila, P., Akerblom, H. K., Isoaho, R., Kauppila, E., and Koivisto, M. (1972) Elimination and Metabolic Effects of Ethanol in Mother, Fetus and Newborn Infant. *American Journal of Obstetrics and Gynecology* **112**: 387–93.

Ijaiya, K., Schwenk, A., and Gladtke, E. (1977) Missbildungen bei Kindern von Alkoholikerinnen (Malformations in Children of Women Alcoholics). *Schwestern Revue* 15: 20.

Ilberg, G. (1904) Sociale Psychiatrie (Social Psychiatry). *Monatsschrift Soziale Medecin* 1: 321.

Illich, I. (1981) *Limits to Medicine: Medical Nemesis*. Harmondsworth: Pelican Books.

—— (1983) *Gender*. London: Marion Boyers.

Illingworth, R. S. (1980) *The Development of the Infant and Young Child* Edinburgh: Churchill Livingstone.

Inglis, B. (1983) *The Diseases of Civilisation*. London: Granada.

Iosub, S., Bingol, N., and Fuchs, M. (1975) Maternal Alcoholism. *Pediatric Research* 9: 284.

Iosub, S., Fuchs, M., Bingol, N., and Gromisch, D. S. (1981) Fetal Alcohol Syndrome Revisited. *Pediatrics* 68 (4): 475–79.

Jarnfelt-Samsioe, A., Samsioe, G., Waldenstrom, J., and Eriksson, B. (1984) Gamma-glutamyltransferase in Normal Pregnancy (letter). *Clinical Chemistry* 30 (5): 807–08.

Jellinek, E. M. and Jolliffe, N. (1940) Effect of Alcohol on the Individual: Review of the Literature of 1939. *Quarterly Journal of Studies on Alcohol* 1: 110–181.

Jessor, R., Graves, R. D., Hanson, R. C., and Jessor, S. L. (1968) *Society, Personality and Deviant Behaviour: A Study of a Tri-Ethnic Community*. New York: Holt, Rhinehart and Winston.

Jewett, J. F. (1976) Committee on Maternal Welfare: Alcoholism and Ruptured Uterus. *New England Journal of Medicine* 294: 335.

Joffe, J. M. (1969) *Prenatal Determinants of Behaviour*. International Series of Monographs in Experimental Psychology vol. 7. Oxford: Pergamon.

Johnson, K. G. (1979) FAS: Rhinorrhea, Persistent Otitis Media, Choanal Stenosis, Hydroplastic Sphenoids and Ethmoid. *Rocky Mountain Medical Journal* 76: 64.

Johnson, P. J. (1984) Sex Hormones and the Liver. *Clinical Science* 66 (4): 369–76.

Jones, B. M. and Jones, M. K. (1976) Alcohol Effects in Women During Menstrual Cycle. *Annals New York Academy Science* 273: 576.

—— (1976) Women and Alcohol: Intoxication, Metabolism and the Menstrual Cycle. In M. Greenblatt and M. A. Schuckit (eds) *Alcohol Problems in Women and Children*. New York: Grune & Stratton.

Jones, K. L. (1975a) Aberrant Neuronal Migration in the Fetal Alcohol Syndrome. *Birth Defects* 11: 131.

—— (1975b) The Fetal Alcohol Syndrome. *Addictive Diseases* 2: 79.

—— (1977) Fetal Alcohol Syndrome. In J. L. Rementeria (ed.) *Drug Abuse in Pregnancy and Neonatal Effects*. St. Louis: C. V. Mosby.

Jones, K. L. and Chernoff, G. F. (1978) Drugs and Chemicals Associated with Intrauterine Growth Deficiency. *Journal of Reproductive Medicine* 21: 365.

Jones, K. L., Hanson, J. W., and Smith, D. W. (1978) Palpebral Fissure Size in Newborn Infants. *Journal of Pediatrics* **92**: 787.

Jones, K. L. and Smith, D. W. (1973) Recognition of the Fetal Alcohol Syndrome in Early Infancy. *Lancet* **2**: 999–1001.

Jones, K. L. and Smith, D. W. (1974) Offspring of Chronic Alcoholic Women. *Lancet* **2**: 349.

—— (1975) The Fetal Alcohol Syndrome. List of Abnormalities. *Teratology* **12**: 1–10.

—— (1978) Effects of Alcohol on the Fetus. *New England Journal of Medicine* **298**: 55.

Jones, K. L., Smith, D. W., and Hanson, J. W. (1976) The Fetal Alcohol Syndrome: Clinical Delineation. *Annals New York Academy of Science* **273**: 130.

Jones, K. L., Smith, D. W., and Streissguth, A. P. (1974) Incidence of the FAS in Offspring of Chronically Alcoholic Women. *Pediatric Resident* **84**: 440.

Jones, K. L., Smith, D. W., Streissguth, A. P., and Myrianthopoulos, N. C. (1974) Outcome in Offspring of Chronic Alcoholic Women. *Lancet* **1**: 1076–78.

Jones, K. L., Smith, D. A., Ulleland, C. N., and Streissguth, A. P. (1973) Pattern of Malformation in Offspring of Alcoholic Mothers. *Lancet* June: 1267–71.

Josselyn, I. M. (1978) *Psychosocial Development of Children: Second Edition*. New York: Family Service Association of America.

Jouppila, P., Huikko, M., and Järvinen, P. A. (1970) Effect of Ethyl Alcohol on Urinary Excretion of Noradrenaline and Adrenaline in Patients: Threatened Premature Delivery. *Acta Obstet. Gynecol. Scandinavica* **49**: 359.

Joynt, R. (1974) Mental Retardation and Alcoholism. *Pointer* **21**: 76.

Judges (1952) *The Holy Bible*. London: Collins.

Kaij, L. (1960) *Alcoholism in Twins*. Stockholm: Almqvist & Wiksell.

Kaij, L. and Dock, J. (1975) Grandsons of Alcoholics: A Test of Sex Linked Transmission of Alcohol Abuse. *Archives of General Psychiatry* **32**: 1379–81.

Kalant, O. J. (ed.) (1980) *Research Advances in Alcohol and Drug Problems, Volume 5: Alcohol and Drug Problems in Women*. New York and London: Plenum Press.

Kalton, G. (1966) *Introduction to Statistical Ideas: For Social Scientists*. London: Chapman & Hall.

Kamen, B. and Kamen, S. (1981) *The Kamen Plan for Total Nutrition During Pregnancy*. New York: Appleton-Century-Crofts.

Kaminski, M. (1979) Response to Questions on Alcohol Consumption in Pregnant Women and the Outcome of Pregnancy. *Alcoholism: Clinical and Experimental Research* **3**: 92.

Kaminski, M., Franc, M., Lebouvier, M., Du Mazaubrun, C., and Rumeau-

Rouquette, C. (1981) Moderate Alcohol Use and Pregnancy Outcome. *Neurobehavioral Toxicology and Teratology* 3: 173–81.

Kaminski, M., Rumeau-Rouquette, C., and Schwartz, D. (1976) Consommation d'Alcool chez les Femmes Enceintes et Issue de la Grossesse. *Revue Epidémiologie Santé, Publi* 24: 27–40. English Translation by Little, R. E. and Schinzel, A. (1978) Alcohol Consumption in Pregnant Women and the Outcome of Pregnancy. *American Journal of Public Health* 57: 2071–75.

—— (1978a) Alcohol Consumption in Pregnant Women and the Outcome of Pregnancy. *Alcoholism: Clinical and Experimental Research* 2 (2): 155–63.

—— (1978b) Effects of Alcohol on the Fetus. *New England Journal of Medicine* 298: 55.

Kandel, D. B. (ed.) (1978) *Longitudinal Research on Drug Use.* London: Halstead (Wiley).

Kartun, D. (1982) Babies on the Bottle. *The Times Health Supplement* 19 February.

Keller, M. (1955) How Alcohol Affects the Body. *(Popular Pamphlet No. 3)* New Brunswick: Rutgers Center of Alcohol Studies.

Kennedy, I. (1983) *The Unmasking of Medicine.* London: Granada.

Kerr, C. (1977) *Sex for Women.* New York: Grove Press.

Kesaniemi, Y. A. (1974) 'Studies in the Ethanol Combined Galactose Elimination Test with Special Reference to Pregnancy.' Dissertation, University of Helsinki.

—— (1974) Ethanol and Acetaldehyde in the Milk and Peripheral Blood of Lactating Women after Ethanol Administration. *Journal of Obstetrics and Gynaecology British Commonwealth* 81: 84.

Kesaniemi, Y. A., Kurppa, K. O., and Husman, K. R. H. (1974) Ethanol-Combined Galactose Tolerance Test in Healthy Pregnant Women and the Effect of a High-Protein Diet. *Journal of Obstetrics and Gynaecology British Commonwealth* 80: 344.

Kessel, N. (1977) The Fetal Alcohol Syndrome from the Public Health Standpoint. *Health Trends* 8: 86–9.

—— (1980) Personal communication.

Keynes, J. M. (1910–11) Influence of Parental Alcoholism. *Journal of the Royal Statistical Society* 74: 339–45.

Khan, A., Bader, J. L., Hoy, G. R., and Sinks, L. F. (1979) Hepatoblastoma in Child with FAS. *Lancet* 1: 1403.

Kiebooms, L. (1979) Abortus en het Foetale Alcohol Syndroom (Abortion and the FAS). *South African Medical Journal* 55: 155.

Kilich, S. and Plant, M. A. (1981) Regional Variations in Levels of Alcohol Related Problems in Britain. *British Journal of Addiction* 76: 47–62; erratum note (1982) 77: 211.

Kim, S. S. and Hodgkinson, R. (1976) Acute Ethanol Intoxication and its Prolonged Effect on a Full-term Neonate. *Anaesthetic and Analgesics Current Research* 55: 602.

144   *Women, Drinking, and Pregnancy*

King, J. C. and Fabro, S. (1983) Alcohol Consumption and Cigarette Smoking: Effect on Pregnancy. *Clinical Obstetrics and Gynecology* 26 (2): 437–48.

Kirkpatrick, S. E., Pitlick, P. T., Hirschklau, M. J., and Friedman, W. F. (1976) Acute Effects of Maternal Ethanol Infusion on Fetal Cardiac Performance. *American Journal of Obstetrics and Gynecology* 126: 1034–37.

Kitzinger, S. (1962) *The Experience of Childbirth*. London: Gollancz.

—— (1977a) *Education and Counselling for Childbirth*. London: Baillière Tindall.

—— (1977b) *Giving Birth: Emotions in Childbirth*. New York: Schocken Books.

—— (1979a) *Birth at Home*. Oxford: Oxford University Press.

—— (1979b) *The Experience of Breastfeeding*. Harmondsworth: Penguin.

—— (1979c) *The Good Birth Guide*. London: Fontana.

—— (1980) *Pregnancy and Childbirth*.

—— (1981) *Women as Mothers*. Glasgow: Collins.

Klassen, R. W. and Persaud, T. V. N. (1976) Experimental Studies on the Influence of Male Alcoholism on Pregnancy and Progeny. *Experimental Pathology* 12: 38.

Kline, J., Shrout, P., Stein, Z., Susser, M., and Warburton, D. (1980) Drinking During Pregnancy and Spontaneous Abortion. *Lancet* July 26: 176–80.

Knightly, P., Evans, H., Potter, E., and Wallace, M. (1979) *Suffer the Children: The Story of Thalidomide*. London: André Deutsch.

Kolata G. B. (1981) Fetal Alcohol Advisory Debated. *Science* 214: 642–45.

Kollerstrom, N. (1982) *Lead on the Brain*. London: Wildwood House.

Koranyi, G. (1978) Embryopathia Alcoholica (Alcoholic Embryopathy). *Alkohologia* 9: 70.

Kotzin, M. (1977) Fetal Alcohol Syndrome. *Media Methods* 14: 23.

Kricka, L. J. and Clark, P. M. S. (1979) *Biochemistry of Alcohol and Alcoholism*. Chichester: John Wiley.

Kruse, J. (1984) Alcohol Use During Pregnancy. *American Family Physician* 29 (4): 199–203.

Kumar, S. P. (1982) Fetal Alcohol Syndrome Mechanisms and Teratogenesis. *Annals of Clinical and Laboratory Science* 12 (4): 254–57.

Kupfermann, J. (1979) *The Mstaken Body: A Fresh Perspective on the Women's Movement*. London: Granada.

Kuzma, J. and Kissinger, D. G. (1981) Patterns of Alcohol and Cigarette Use in Pregnancy. *Neurobehavioral Toxicology and Teratology* 3: 211–21.

Kuzma, J. and Sokol, R. (1982) Maternal Drinking Behavior and Decreased Intra Uterine Growth. *Alcoholism: Clinical and Experimental Research* 6 (3): 396–402.

Lamache, A. (1967) Reflexions sur la Descendance des Alcooliques. *Bulletin d'Academie Nationale de Médicine* 151: 517–21.

Landesman-Dwyer, S. (1982) Maternal Drinking and Pregnancy Outcome. *Applied Research Mental Retardation* 3 (3): 241–63.

Landesman-Dwyer, S., Keler, L. S., and Streissguth, A. P. (1978) Naturalistic Observations of Newborns: Effects of Maternal Alcohol Intake. *Alcoholism: Clinical and Experimental Research* 2 (2): 171–77.

Landesman-Dwyer, S., Ragozin, A. S., and Little, R. E. (1981) Behavioural Correlates of Prenatal Alcohol Exposure: A Four Year Follow-up. *Neurobehavioral Toxicology and Teratology* 3 (2): 187–93.

Lanson, L. (1977) *From Woman to Woman.* Harmondsworth: Pelican Books.

Larsson, G. (1983) Prevention of Fetal Alcohol Effects. *Acta Obstetrica Gynecologie Scandinavica* 62: 171–78.

Larsson, G., Ottenblad, C., Hagenfeldt, L., Larsson, A., and Forsgren, M. (1983) Evaluation of Serum Gamma-glutamyl Transferase as a Screening Method for Excessive Alcohol Consumption during Pregnancy. *American Journal of Obstetrics and Gynecology* 147 (6): 654–57.

Leeson, J. and Gray, J. (1978) *Women and Medicine.* London: Tavistock.

Lefkowitch, J. H., Rushton, A. R., and Feng-Chen, K. C. (1983) Hepatic Fibrosis in Fetal Alcohol Syndrome. Pathologic Similarities to Adult Alcoholic Liver Disease. *Gastroenterology* 85 (4): 951–57.

LeFrancois, C. (1984) Fetal Alcohol Syndrome. Maternal Alcohol Ingestion: Serious Consequences for the Fetus. *Vt. Registered Nurse* April: 3–5.

Lele, A. S. (1982) Fetal Alcohol Syndrome: Other Effects of Alcohol on Pregnancy. *New York State Journal of Medicine* July: 1225–227.

Lemoine, P., Harronsseau, H., Borteyru, J. P., and Menuet, J. C. (1968) Les Enfants De Parents Alcooliques: Anomalies Observées A propos 127 Cas. *Ouest Médicale* 25: 476–82.

Lenz, W. (1966) Malformations Caused by Drugs in Pregnancy. *American Journal of Diseases of Childhood* 112: 99.

(Letter) (1978) Effects of Alcohol on the Fetus. *New England Journal of Medicine* 298 (1): 55–6.

Lewis, D. D. (1983) Alcohol and Pregnancy Outcome. *Midwives Chronical* 96 (1151): 420–22.

Lieber, C. S. (1984) To Drink (Moderately) or Not to Drink? (Editorial). *New England Journal of Medicine* 29 March 13: 846–48.

Lightfoot, E. C., Keeling, B., and Wilton, K. M. (1982) Characteristics Distinguishing High-Anxious and Med/Low-Anxious Women During Pregnancy. *Journal of Psychosomatic Research* 26 (3): 345–50.

Lim, K. B. and Hawkins, D. F. (1983) Drugs in Pregnancy. *Midwife Health Visitor Community Nurse* 19 (12): 458–63.

Lindenschmidt, R. R. and Persaud, T. V. N. (1980) Effects of Ethanol and Nicotine in the Pregnant Rat. *Research Communications in Chemical Pathology and Pharmacology* 271: 195–98.

Linn, S., Schoenbaum, S. C., Mouson, R. R., Rosner, B., Stubblefield, P. G., and Ryan, K. J. (1982) No Association Between Coffee Consump-

146   *Women, Drinking, and Pregnancy*

tion and Adverse Outcomes of Pregnancy. *New England Journal of Medicine* **306**: 141–45.

—— (1983) Lack of Association Between Contraceptive Usage and Congenital Malformations in Offspring. *American Journal of Obstetrics and Gynecology*, 15 December: 147 (8): 923–28.

Little, R. E. (1976) Alcohol Consumption in Pregnancy as Reported to the Obstetrician and to an Independent Interviewer. *Annals of the New York Academy of Sciences* **273**: 588–92.

—— (1977) Moderate Alcohol Use During Pregnancy and Decreased Infant Birth Weight. *American Journal of Public Health* **67** (12): 1154–156.

—— (1979) Drinking During Pregnancy: Implications for Public Health. *Alcohol Health and Research World* **4**: 1.

—— (1981) Epidemiologic and Experimental Studies in Drinking and Pregnancy: The State of the Art. *Neurobehavioral Toxicology and Teratology* **3**: 163–67.

Little, R. E., Graham, J. M. Jnr., and Samson, H. H. (1982) Fetal Alcohol Effects in Humans and Animals. In B. Stimmel (ed.) *The Effects of Maternal Alcohol and Drug Abuse in the Newborn* **1** (3/4): 103–25 New York: Haworth Press.

Little, R. E., Grathwohl, H. L., Streissguth, A. P., and McIntyre, C. (1981) Public Awareness and Knowledge about the Risks of Drinking During Pregnancy in Multnomah County, Oregon. *American Journal of Public Health* **71**: 312–14.

Little, R. E., Schultz. F. A., and Mandell, W. (1976) Drinking During Pregnancy. *Journal of Studies on Alcohol* **37** (3): 375–79.

Little, R. E. and Streissguth, A. P. (1978) Drinking During Pregnancy in Alcoholic Women. *Alcoholism: Clinical and Experimental Research* **2**: 179–83.

—— (1981) Fetal Alcohol Effects: Impact and Prevention. *Canadian Medical Association Journal* **125**: 159–64.

—— (1982) *Alcohol: Pregnancy and the Fetal Alcohol Syndrome. Unit 5 of Alcohol Use and Its Medical Consequences: A Comprehensive Teaching Program for Biomedical Education.* Project Cork of Dartmouth Medical School. Maryland: Milner-Fenwick MD.

Little, R. E., Streissguth, A. P., Barr, H. M. and Herman, C. S. (1980) Decreased Birthweight in Infants of Alcoholic Women Who Abstained During Pregnancy. *Journal of Pediatrics* **96**: 974–76.

Little, R. E., Streissguth, A. P., and Guzinski, G. M. (1980) Prevention of Fetal Alcohol Syndrome: A Model Program. *Alcoholism: Clinical and Experimental Research* **4** (2): 185–89.

Little, R. E., Streissguth, A. P., and Page, E. (1979) Techniques for Recruiting Special Types of Persons for Research: Pitfalls and Successes in Enlisting Recovered Alcoholic Women. *Public Health Reports* **94**: 332–35.

Little, R. E., Streissguth, A. P., Guzinski, G. M., Grathwohl, H. L.,

Blumhagen, J. M., and McIntyre, C. E. (1983) Change in Obstetrician Advice Following a Two Year Community Educational Program on Alcohol Use and Pregnancy. *American Journal of Obstetrics and Gynecology* 146: 23–8.

Llewellyn-Jones, D. (1982) *Everywoman: A Gynaecological Guide for Life.* London: Faber & Faber.

—— (1983) *The A-Z of Women's Health.* Oxford: Oxford University Press.

London Feminist History Group (1983) *The Sexual Dynamics of History.* London: Pluto Press.

Long, J. F. (1879) Use and Abuse of Alcohol. *North Carolina Medical Journal* 4: 85–98.

Loser, U. and Majewski, F. (1977) Type and Frequency of Cardiac Defects in Embryo-Fetal Alcohol Syndrome: Report of 16 Cases. *British Heart Journal* 39: 1374–379.

Lowry, R. B. (1977) The Klippel-Feil Anomology as Part of the Fetal Alcohol Syndrome. *Teratology* 16: 53–6.

Lund, C. (1976) A Reliable and Inexpensive Device for Measuring Head-Turning. *Journal of Experimental Child Psychology* 21: 361–6.

McAllister, P. (ed.) (1982) *Reweaving the Web of Life.* Philadelphia, Pa.: New Society Publishers.

McCandless, P. (1984) 'Curses of Civilization': Insanity and Drunkenness in Victorian Britain. *British Journal of Addiction* 79: 49–58.

McCarty, D. and Ewing, J. A. (1983) Alcohol Consumption While Viewing Alcoholic Beverage Advertising. *International Journal of Addiction* 18 October (7): 1019–27.

MacDowell, E. C. and Vicari, E. M. (1917) On the Growth and Fecundity of Alcoholized Rats. *Proceedings National Academy of Science* 3: 577–79.

MacFarlane, J. A. (1980) *Child Health.* London: Grant McIntyre.

Mackay, J. R. (1961) Clinical Observations on Adolescent Problem Drinking. *Quarterly Journal of Studies on Alcohol* 22: 124–34.

McKeown, T. (1982) *The Role of Medicine.* Oxford: Basil Blackwell.

Mackie, L. and Pattullo, P. (1977) *Women at Work.* London: Tavistock.

MacLennan, A. (ed.) (1976) *Women: Their Use of Alcohol and Other Legal Drugs.* Toronto: Addiction Research Foundation of Ontario.

Macy, C. and Falkener, F. (1979) *Pregnancy and Birth: Pleasures and Problems.* London: Harper & Row.

Majewski, F. (1981) Alcohol Embryopathy: Some Facts and Speculations About Pathogenesis. *Neurobehavioral Toxicology and Teratology* 3: 129–44.

Mann, L. I., Bhakthavathsalan, A., Liu, M., and Makowski, P. (1975) Placental Transport of Alcohol and Its Effect on Maternal and Fetal Acid-Base Balance. *American Journal of Obstetrics and Gynecology* 122: 837–44.

—— (1976) Effect of Alcohol on Fetal Cerebral Function and Metabolism. *American Journal of Obstetrics and Gynecology* 122: 845–51.

Marbury, M. C., Linn, S., Monson, R., Schoenbaum, S., Stubblefield, P. G., and Ryan, K. J. (1983) The Association of Alcohol Consumption with Outcome of Pregnancy. *American Journal of Public Health* **73** (10): 1165–168.

Marcus, M. (1981) *A Taste for Pain: On Masochism and Female Sexuality.* London: Souvenir Press.

Margolin, F. G. (1977) Fetal Alcohol Syndrome: Report of a Case. *Journal of the American Obstetrical Association* **77**: 50/99–52/101.

Marsh, C. (1982) *The Survey Method: The Contribution of Surveys to Sociological Explanation.* London: Allen & Unwin.

Marsh, D. (1980) *The Welfare State.* London: Longman.

Marsteller, P. and Karnchanapee, K. (1980) The Use of Women in the Advertising of Distilled Spirits 1956–79. *Journal of Psychedelic Drugs* **12**: 1–12.

Martin, D. C., Martin, J. C., Streissguth, A. P., and Lund, C. A. (1979) Sucking Frequency and Amplitude in Newborns as a Function of Maternal Drinking and Smoking. In M. Gallanter (ed.) *Currents in Alcoholism*, Vol. V. New York: Grune and Stratton.

Martin, J. (1977) The Fetal Alcohol Syndrome: Recent Findings. *Alcohol Health and Research World* **1** (3): 8–12.

Martin, J. C., Martin, D. C., Lund, C. A., and Streissguth, A. P. (1977) Maternal Alcohol Ingestion and Cigarette Smoking and Their Effects on Newborn Conditioning. *Alcoholism: Clinical and Experimental Research* **1**: 243–47.

Martin, J. C., Martin, D. C., Sigman, G., and Ladow, B. (1977) Offspring Survival, Development and Operant Performance Following Maternal Ethanol Consumption. *Developmental Psychobiology* **10**: 435–46.

Mau, G. and Netter, P. (1974) Kaffee und Alkoholkonsum Risikofactoren in der Schwangerschaft? (Are Coffee and Alcohol Consumption Risk Factors in Pregnancy?). *Geburtschulfe Frauenheilkd* **34**: 1018–22.

Maury, E. A. (1976) *Wine is the Best Medicine.* London: Souvenir Press.

Mayer, J. and Black, R. (1977) The Relationship between Alcoholism and Child/Abuse/Neglect. In F. A. Seixas (ed.) *Currents in Alcoholism* **2**: 429–44. New York: Grune & Stratton.

Mayfield, D., McLeod, D., and Ha, P. (1974) The CAGE Questionnaire: Validation of a New Alcoholism Screening Instrument. *American Journal of Psychiatry* **131** (10): 1121–123.

Melville, A. and Johnson, C. (1982) *Cured to Death.* London: Secker & Warburg.

Mena, M. R., Albornoz, C., Puente, M., and Moreno, C. (1980) Sindrome Fetal Alcoholico. Estudio de 19 Casos Clinicos. *Revisita Chilena de Pediatria* **51**: 414–23.

Mendelson, J. W. (1978) The Fetal Alcohol Syndrome (letter). *New England Journal of Medicine* **299** (10): 556.

Midanik, L. (1982a) The Validity of Self-Reported Alcohol Consumption and Alcohol Problems: A Literature Review. *British Journal of Addiction*

77 (4): 357-82.
—— (1982b) Over Reports of Recent Alcohol Consumption in a Clinical Population: A Validity Study. *Drug and Alcohol Dependence* **9**: 101-10.
Miller, C. and Swift, K. (1981) *The Handbook of Non-Sexist Writing.* London: The Women's Press.
Miller, J. B. (1978) *Towards a New Psychology of Women.* London: Allen Lane.
Mitchell, J. (1981) *Women's Estate.* Harmondsworth: Pelican Books.
Moghissi, K. S. (1978) Maternal Nutrition in Pregnancy. *Clinical Obstetrics and Gynecology* **21** (2): 297-310.
Montague, A. (1965) *Life Before Birth.* New York: Signet.
Morelock, S., Hingson, R., Kayne, H., Dooling, E., Zuckerman, B., Day, N., Alpert, J. J., and Flowerdew, G. (1982) Bendectin and Fetal Development: A Study at Boston City Hospital. *American Journal of Obstetrics and Gynecology* **142** (2): 209-13.
Morris, C. (1751) *Observations on the Past and Present Growth and the Present State of London.* London: A. Millar.
Morris, J. B. and Hird, M. D. (1981) A Neuro-Developmental Infant Screening Programme Undertaken by Health Visitors – Preliminary Report. *Health Bulletin* **39** (4): 236-50.
Morris, M. B. and Weinstein, L. (1981) Caffeine and the Fetus: Is Trouble Brewing? *American Journal of Obstetrics and Gynecology* **140** (6): 607-10.
Morrison, A. B. and Maykut, M. O. (1979) Potential Adverse Effects of Maternal Alcohol Ingestion on the Developing Fetus and Their Sequelae in the Infant and Child. *Canadian Medical Journal* **120** (7): 826-28.
Morrison, J. R. and Stewart, M. A. (1973) Evidence of Polygenetic Inheritance in the Hyperactive Child Syndrome. *American Journal of Psychiatry* **130**: 791-92.
—— (1971) A Family Study of the Hyperactive Child Syndrome. *Biological Psychiatry* **3**: 189-95.
Muir Gray, J. A. (1979) *Man Against Disease.* Oxford: Oxford University Press.
Mukherjee, A. and Hodges, G. (1982) How Drink Can Harm Your Unborn Baby. *The Sunday Times* 14 November.
Mulvihill, J. J., Klimas, J., Stokes, D. C., and Risemberg, H. M. (1976) Fetal Alcohol Syndrome: Seven New Cases. *American Journal of Obstetrics and Gynecology* **125**: 937.
Murai, N. (1966) Effect of Maternal Medication During Pregnancy upon Behavioural Development of Offspring. *Tohoku Journal of Experimental Medicine* **89**: 265.
Murray-Lyon, I. M., Barrison, I. G., Wright, J. T., Morris, N., and Gordon, M. (1980) Alcohol Abuse in Pregnancy: A Problem (letter). *Lancet* 20 December: 27.
National Broadcasting Company (1976) Fetal Alcohol Syndrome. *Landers Film Reviews* Sept/Oct **21**: 13.

150   Women, Drinking, and Pregnancy

National Council for Women in the UK (1980) *The Fetal Alcohol Syndrome* (Report of the Working Party on Alcohol Problems). London.

National Institute for Alcohol and Alcohol Abuse Workshop (1977) *The FAS and Other Effects on Offspring*. NIAAA Sponsored Workshop, February 1977.

Neugut, R. H. (1982) Fetal Alcohol Syndrome: How Good is the Evidence? *Neurobehavioral-Toxicology and Teratology* 4 (6): 593–94.

Newton, J. L., Ryan, M. P., and Walkowitz, J. R. (1983) *Sex and Class in Women's History*. London: Routledge & Kegan Paul.

Nice, L. B. (1912) Comparative Studies on the Effects of Alcohol, Nicotine, Tobacco Smoke and Caffeine on White Mice. *Journal of Experimental Zoology* 12: 133–52.

—— (1917) Further Observations on the Effects of Alcohol on White Mice. *American Naturalist* 51: 596–607.

Nie, N. H., Hull, C. H., Jenkins, J. G., Steinbrenner, K., and Bent, D. H. (1975) *Statistical Package for the Social Scientist: Second Edition*. New York: McGraw-Hill.

Nilsson, L. (1981) *A Child is Born*. London: Faber & Faber.

Nin, A. (1982) *A Woman Speaks*. London: W. H. Allen.

Noonon, J. A. (1976) Congenital Heart Disease in the Fetal Alcohol Syndrome. *American Journal of Cardiology* 36: 160.

—— (1976) Congenital Heart Disease in the Fetal Alcohol Syndrome. *American Journal of Obstetrics and Gynecology* 125: 937–41.

Norusis, M. J. (1983) *SPSS X: Introductory Statistics Guide*. New York: McGraw-Hill.

Nylander, I. (1960) Children of Alcoholic Fathers. *Acta Paediatrica Scandinavica* 49 (1): 134.

Nylander. I and Rydelius, P. A. (1983) A Comparison between Children of Alcoholic Fathers from Excellent versus Poor Social Conditions. *Acta Paediatrica Scandinavica* 71 (5): 809–13.

Oakley, A. (1972) *Sex, Gender and Society*. London: Temple Smith.

—— (1979) *Becoming a Mother*. Oxford: Martin Robertson.

—— (1980) *Women Confined: Towards a Sociology of Childbirth*. Oxford: Martin Robertson.

—— (1981) *From Here to Maternity: Becoming a Mother*. Harmondsworth: Pelican Books.

—— (1982) *Subject Women*. London: Fontana.

O'Conner, J. (1978) *The Young Drinkers*. London: Tavistock.

Olegard, R. and Aronson, M. (1982) Alkohol och Graviditet-Foltderna for Barnet. (English Summary.) *Nordisk Medicin* 97 (1): 6–8.

Olegard, R., Aronsson, M., Carlsson, C., Johansson, P. R., Kyllerman, M., Sabel, K. G., and Sandin, B. (1977) Alcohol in Pregnancy. *Lakartidningen* 74: 3074.

Olegard, R., Sabel, K. G., Aronsson, M., Sandin, B., Johansson, P. R., Carlsson, C., Kyllerman, M., Iversen, K., and Hrbek, A. (1979) Effects on the Child of Alcohol Abuse During Pregnancy. *Acta Paediatrica Scandinavica Supplement* **275**: 112-21.

Olsen, J., Rachootin, P., and Schiodt, A. V. (1983) Alcohol Use, Conception Time and Birth Weight. *Journal of Epidemiology and Community Health* **37**: 63-5.

Olsen, J., Rachootin, P., Schiodt, A. V., and Damsbo, N. (1983) Tobacco Use, Alcohol Consumption and Infertility. *International Journal of Epidemiology* **12** (2): 179-84.

O'Neill, P. (1983) *Health Crisis 2000*. Oxford: The Alden Press.

O'Shea, K. S. and Kaufmann, H. (1979) The Teratogenic Effect of Acetaldehyde: Implications for the Study of the Fetal Alcohol Syndrome. *Journal of Anatomy* **128** (1): 65-76.

Ouellette, E. M. and Rosett, H. L. (1976) A Pilot Prospective Study of the Fetal Alcohol Syndrome at the Boston City Hospital (2) The Infants. *Annals of the New York Academy of Science* **273**: 123-28.

Ouellette, E. M., Rosett, H. L., Rosman, N. P., and Weiner, L. (1977) Adverse Effects on Offspring of Maternal Alcohol Abuse During Pregnancy. *New England Journal of Medicine* **297**: 528.

Palmer, R. H., Ouellette, E. M., Warner, L., and Leichtman, S. R. (1974) Congenital Malformations in Offspring of a Chronic Alcoholic Mother. *Pediatrics* **53**: 490-94.

Pap, A. G., Dishlow, V. D., and Guttman, L. B. (1970) The Cardiovascular System During Pregnancy. *International Journal Obstetrics and Gynaecology* **8**: 337.

Papara-Nicholson, D. and Telford, I. R. (1957) Effects of Alcohol on Reproduction and Fetal Development in the Guinea Pig. *Anatomical Record* **127**: 438.

Patrick, D. L. and Scambler, G. (eds) (1982) *Sociology As Applied to Medicine*. London: Cassell.

Pearl, R. (1916) The Effect of Parental Alcoholism (and Certain Other Drug Intoxications) Upon the Progeny in the Domestic Fowl. *Proceedings of the National Academy of Science* **2**: 675.

—— (1917) The Experimental Modification of Germ Cells. *Journal Experimental Zoology* **22** (125) (186): 241-310.

Peck, D. (1982) Some Determining Factors. In M. A. Plant (ed) *Drinking and Problem Drinking*. London: Junction Books.

Perlin, M. J. and Simon, K. J. (1978) The Etiology Prevalence and Effects of Drug Use During Pregnancy. *Contemporary Drug Problems* Fall: 311-26.

Pernanen, K. (1974) Validity of Survey Data on Alcohol Use. In R. J. Gibbens, Y. Israel, H. Kalant, R. E. Popham, W. Schmidt, and R. G. Smart (eds) *Alcohol and Drug Problems*. New York: Wiley.

Pierog, S., Chandavasu, O., and Wexler, I. (1977) Withdrawal Symptoms in Infant with Fetal Alcohol Syndrome. *Journal of Pediatrics* **9** (2): 64-7.

—— (1979) The Fetal Alcohol Syndrome: Some Maternal Characteristics.

152 Women, Drinking, and Pregnancy

International Journal of Gynaecology and Obstetrics 16: 412–15.

Pihl, R. O., Marinier, R., Lapp, J., and Drake, H. (1982) Psychotropic Drug Use by Women: Characteristics of High Consumers. International Journal of the Addictions 17 (2): 259–69.

Pilstrom, L. and Keissling, K. H. (1967) Effect of Ethanol on the Growth and on the Liver and Brain Mitochondrial Functions of the Offspring of Rats. Acta Pharmacologia et Toxicologia 25: 225–32.

Plant, M. A. (1975) Drugtakers in an English Town. London: Tavistock.

—— (1979) Drinking Careers. London: Tavistock.

—— (1981) Drugs in Perspective. London: Hodder & Stoughton.

—— (ed.) (1982) Drinking and Problem Drinking. London: Junction Books.

Plant, M. A. and Miller, T. I. (1977) Disguised and Undisguised Questionnaires Compared: Two Alternative Approaches to Drinking Behaviour Surveys. Social Psychiatry 12: 21–4.

Plant, M. A., Peck, D. F., and Stuart, R. (1982) Self-Reported Drinking Habits and Alcohol-Related Consequences Amongst a Cohort of Scottish Teenagers. British Journal of Addiction 77: 75–90.

—— (1984) The Correlates of Serious Alcohol-Related Consequences and Illicit Drug Use Amongst Scottish Teenagers. British Journal of Addiction 79: 197–200.

Plant, M. L. (1980) Nurse Education: Present Problems and Future Needs. In J. S. Madden, R. Walker, and W. H. Kenyon (eds) Aspects of Alcoholism and Drug Dependence. Tunbridge Wells: Pitman.

—— (1980) The Fetal Alcohol Syndrome. 14th Annual Report of the Glasgow Council on Alcoholism 1: 18–21.

—— (1983) Alcohol Consumption in Pregnancy: Is It Safe? Nursing Mirror October 5: 2–4.

Popham, R. E. (1970) Indirect Methods of Alcoholism Prevalence Estimation: A Critical Review. In R. E. Popham (ed.) Alcohol and Alcoholism. Toronto: Toronto University Press.

Poskitt, E. M. E., Hensey, O. J., and Smith, C. S. (1982) Alcohol, Other Drugs and the Fetus. Developmental Medicine Child Neurolology. 24: 596–602.

Potter, D., Anderson, J., Clarke, J., Coombes, P., Hall, S., Harris, L., Holloway, C. and Walton, T. (eds) (1981) Society and the Social Sciences: An Introduction. London: Routledge & Kegan Paul.

Prager, K., Malin, H., Spiegler, D., Van-Natta, P., and Placek, P.J. (1984) Smoking and Drinking Behavior Before and During Pregnancy of Married Mothers of Live-born Infants and Stillborn Infants. Public Health Report 99 (2): 17–127.

Pratt, O. E. (1980) The Transport of Nutrients into the Brain: The Effects of Alcohol on their Supply and Utilization. In D. Richter (ed.) Addiction and Brain Damage. London: Croom Helm.

—— (1981) Alcohol and the Woman of Childbearing Age – A Public Health Problem. British Journal of Addiction 76: 389–90.

—— (1982) Alcohol and the Developing Fetus. *British Medical Bulletin* 34: 48–52.

Qazi, Q. H. and Masakawa, A. (1976) Altered Sex Ration in Fetal Alcohol Syndrome. *Lancet* 2: 42.

Qazi, Q. H., Madahar, C., Masakawa, A., and McGann, B. (1979a) Chromosome Abnormality in a Patient with Fetal Alcohol Syndrome. In M. Galanter (ed.) *Currents in Alcoholism Vol. 5 Biomedical Issues and Clinical Effects of Alcoholism.* New York: Grune & Stratton.

Qazi, Q. H., Masakawa, A., Milman, D., McGann, D., Chua, A., and Haller, J. (1979b) Renal Anomalies in Fetal Alcohol Syndrome. *Pediatrics* 63 (6): 886–89.

Randall, C. (1977) Teratogenic Effects of in Utero Ethanol Exposure. In K. Bloom (ed.) *Alcohol and Opiates: Neurochemical and Behavioral Mechanisms.* New York: Academic Press.

Randall, C. L. and Noble, E. P. (1980) Alcohol Abuse and Fetal Growth and Development. In N. K. Mello (ed.) *Advances in Substance Abuse. Behavioral and Biological Research: A Research Annual.* Greenwich Connecticut: JAI Press.

Randall, C. L. and Taylor, W. J. (1979) Prenatal Ethanol Exposure in Mice: Teratogenic Effects. *Teratology* 19: 305–12.

Randall, C. L., Lochry, E. A., and Sutker, P. B. (1981) Effects of Acute Alcohol Exposure During Selected Days of Gestation in C_3H Mice. *Teratology* 23: 57A.

Rane, A., Von Bahr, C., Orrenius, S., and Sjoqvist, F. (1973) Drug Metabolism in the Human Fetus. In L. O. Boreus (ed.) *Fetal Pharmacology.* New York: Raven Press.

Rasmussen, B. B. and Christensen, N. (1977) Alcohol and Fetal Damage. *Ugester Laeger* 140 (6): 282–84.

Ratcliffe, M. L. (1979) Catch a Woman Customer. *Supermarketing* 30 March: 6–7.

Rayburn, W., Wible-Kant, J., and Bledsoe, P. (1982) Changing Trends in Drug Use During Pregnancy. *Journal of Reproductive Medicine* September: 27: 9.

Registrar General (Scotland) (1984) *1981 Sample Census.* Small Area Tables for the City of Edinburgh: 6.

Renwick, J. H. and Asker, R. L. (1982) The Time Course of Response of Erythrocyte Volume to Ethanol and to its Withdrawal. *Clinical Laboratory Haematology* 4 (3): 325–26.

Rich, A. (1981) *Of Woman Born.* London: Virago.

Richards, J. R. (1982) *The Sceptical Feminist: A Philosophical Enquiry.* Harmondsworth: Pelican Books.

Riley, E. P. and Lochry, E. A. (1982) Genetic Influences in the Etiology of Fetal Alcohol Syndrome. In E. L. Abel (ed.) *Fetal Alcohol Syndrome Vol 3. Animal Studies.* Florida: CRC Press.

Riley, E. P., Lochry, E. A., Shapiro, N. R., and Baldwin, J. (1979) Response

154   *Women, Drinking, and Pregnancy*

Perseveration in Rats Exposed to Alcohol Prenatally. *Pharmacology, Biochemistry Behavior* 10: 255–59.

Rimmer, J. and Chambers, D. S. (1969) Alcoholism: Methodological Considerations in the Study of Family Illness. *American Journal Orthopsychiatry* 39: 760–68.

Robe, L. B., Robe, R. S., and Wilson, P. A. (1979) Maternal Heavy Drinking Related to Delayed Onset of Daughters' Menstruation. *Alcoholism: Clinical and Experimental Research* 3: 192. (Abstract)

Robinovitch, L. G. (1901) Idiot and Imbecile Children: Various Causes of Idiocy and Imbecility: The Relation of Alcoholism in the Parent to Idiocy and Imbecility of the Offspring: A Clinical Study. *Journal of Mental Pathology* 1 (14): 86–95.

—— (1903) Infantile Alcoholism. *Quarterly Journal of Inebriety* 25: 231–36.

Roe, A. (1944–45) The Adult Adjustment of Children of Alcoholic Parents Raised in Foster Homes. *Quarterly Journal of Studies on Alcohol* 5 (3): 378–93.

Roe, A. and Burks, B. (1945) *Adult Adjustment of Foster Children of Alcoholic and Psychotic Parentage and the Influence of the Foster Home.* Memoirs of the Section on Alcohol Studies No 3, New Haven, Conn. Yale Univerisity: 1–164.

Roget, P. M. (1980) *Thesaurus of Synonyms and Antonyms.* London: University Books.

Root, A. W., Reiter, E. O., Andriola, M., and Duckett, G. (1975) Hypothalamic-Pituitary Function in the Fetal Alcohol Syndrome. *The Journal of Pediatrics* 87: 585–88.

Rosett, H. L. (1976) The Effects of Maternal Drinking on Child Development – Introductory Review. Work in Progress on Alcohol. *Annals New York Academy of Science* 273: 115–17.

—— (1980) A Clinical Perspective of the Fetal Alcohol Syndrome. *Alcoholism: Clinical and Experimental Research* 14 (2): 119–22.

Rosett, H. L., Ouellette, E. M., and Weiner, L. (1976) A Pilot Prospective Study of the Fetal Alcohol Syndrome at the Boston City Hospital (1) Maternal Drinking. *Annals of the New York Academy of Science* 273: 118–22.

Rosett, H. L., Ouellette, E. M., Weiner, L., and Owens, E. (1978) Therapy of Heavy Drinking During Pregnancy. *American Journal of Obstetrics and Gynecology* 51: 41.

—— (1977) The Prenatal Clinic: A Site for Alcoholism Prevention and Treatment. In F. A. Seixas (ed.) *Currents in Alcoholism* 1: 419. New York: Grune & Stratton.

Rosett, H. L. and Sander, L. W. (1979) Effects of Drinking on Neonatal Morphology and State Regulation. In G. D. Osofsky (ed.) *Handbook for Infant Development.* New York: John Wiley.

Rosett, H. L. and Weiner, L. (1984) *Alcohol and the Fetus.* New York: Oxford.

Rosett, H. L., Weiner, L., Zuckerman, B., McKinlay, S., and Edelin, K. C. (1980) Reduction of Alcohol Consumption During Pregnancy with Benefits to the Newborn. *Alcoholism: Clinical and Experimental Research* 4 (2): 178–84.

Rosett, H. L., Weiner, L., and Edelin, K. C. (1983) Treatment Experience with Pregnant Problem Drinkers. *Journal of the American Medical Association* 249 (15): 2029–33.

Rosett, H. L., Weiner, L., Lee, A., Zuckerman, B., Dooling, E., and Oppenheimer, E. (1983) Patterns of Alcohol Consumption and Fetal Development. *Journal of the American College of Obstetricians and Gynecologists* 61 (5): 539–46.

Rothman, B. K. (1982) *In Labour: Woman and Power in the Birthplace.* London: Junction Books.

Rouguette, P. C. (1957) *The Influence of Parental Alcohol Toxicomania on the Physical and Mental Development of Young Children.* M. D. Thesis. University of Paris.

Rowbotham, S. (1978) *A New World for Women: Stella Browne – Socialist Feminist.* London: Pluto Press.

—— (1981) *Woman's Consciousness, Man's World.* Harmondsworth: Penguin Books.

Rowe, M. (ed.) (1982) *Spare Rib Reader.* Harmondsworth: Penguin Books.

Rowntree, D. (1981) *Statistics Without Tears.* Harmondsworth: Penguin Books.

Royal College of Physicians (1983) *Health or Smoking?* London: Pitman.

Royal College of Psychiatrists (1979) *Alcohol and Alcoholism.* London: Tavistock.

Rush, B. (1787) *An Enquiry into the Effects of Spiritous Liquors upon the Human Body and their Influence upon the Happiness of Society.* Philadelphia: Thomas Dobson.

—— (1812) *An Inquiry into the Effects of Ardent Spirits upon the Human Body and Mind: With an Account of the Means of Preventing, and of the Remedies for Curing Them.* Boston, Mass.: Manning & Loring.

Russell, M. (1977) Intra Uterine Growth in Infants Born to Women with Alcohol-Related Psychiatric Diagnosis. *Alcoholism: Clinical and Experimental Research* 1: 225–31.

Russianoff, P. (ed.) (1981) *Women in Crisis.* New York: Human Sciences Press.

Rutter, M. (1981) *Maternal Deprivation Reassessed: Second Edition.* Harmondsworth: Penguin Books.

Sanders, D. and Reed, J. (1982) *Kitchen Sink or Swim?* Harmondsworth: Penguin Books.

Saul, P. (1983) Nursing Mirror Midwifery Forum 9. Fetal Alcohol Syndrome. *Nursing Mirror* 157 (14): 4–6.

Saunders, J. B., Wodak, A. D., and Williams, R. (1984) What Determines Susceptibility to Liver Damage from Alcohol? *Journal of the Royal*

156   *Women, Drinking, and Pregnancy*

Society of Medicine March **77** (3): 204–16.

Sayers, J. (1982) *Biological Politics*. London: Tavistock.

Schmidt, D. W. (1972) Analysis of Alcohol Consumption Data: The Use of Consumption Data for Research Purposes. *Report on the Conference on Epidemiology of Drug Dependence. London.* World Health Organisation: 57–66.

Schukit, M. A. (1980) Alcoholism and Genetics: Possible Biological Factors. *Biological Psychiatry* **15**: 437–47.

Schwetz, B. A., Smith F. A., and Staples, R. E. (1978) Teratogenic Potential of Ethanol in Mice, Rats and Rabbits. *Teratology* **18**: 385–92.

Segal, L. (1983) *What is to be Done About the Family?* Harmondsworth: Penguin Books.

Seixas, F. A. (1980) Fetal Alcohol Syndrome and the Year of the Child. *Toxiconamies* **12**: 319–29.

Seppala, M., Raiha, N. C. R., and Tamminen, V. (1971) Ethanol Elimination in a Mother and Her Premature Twins. *Lancet* June: 1188–189.

Shaw, S. (1980) Causes of Increase in Drinking Problems. In Camberwell Council on Alcoholism (eds) *Women and Alcohol*. London: Tavistock.

Shaywitz, S. E., Cohen, D. J., and Shaywitz, B. A. (1980) Behavior and Learning Difficulties in Children of Normal Intelligence Born to Alcoholic Mothers. *Journal of Pediatrics* **96** (6): 978–82.

Shilling, S. and Lalich, N. R. (1984) Maternal Occupation and Industry and the Pregnancy Outcome of US Married Women, 1980. *Public Health Report* **99** (2): 152–61.

Shryock, R. H. (1966) *Medicine in America: Historical Essays*. Baltimore: The Johns Hopkins University Press.

Siegel, S. (1956) *Nonparametric Statistics for the Behavioral Sciences*. London: McGraw-Hill Kogakusha.

Silva, V. A., Laranjeira, R. R., Dolnikoff, M., Grinfeld, H., and Masur, J. (1981) Alcohol Consumption during Pregnancy and Newborn Outcome. *Neurobehavioral Toxicology and Teratology* **3** (2): 169–72.

Silver, H. K., Kempe, C. H., and Bruyn, N. B. (1980) *Handbook of Pediatrics*. Los Altos, Calif.: Lange Medical Publications.

Smart, C. and Smart, B. (eds) (1978) *Women, Sexuality and Social Control*. London: Routledge & Kegan Paul.

Snyder, C. R. (1962) *Culture and Jewish Sobriety: The Ingroup-Outgroup Factor, Culture and Drinking Patterns.* In D. J. Pittman and C. R. Snyder (eds). London: John Wiley.

—— (1978) *Alcohol and the Jews*. Southern Illinois University Press: Arcturus Paperbacks.

Social Services Committee (1980) *Perinatal and Neonatal Mortality*. London: HMSO.

Sokol, R. (1982) Alcohol and Pregnancy: A Clinical Perspective for Laboratory Research. *Substance and Alcohol Actions/Misuse* **3**: 183–6.

Sokol, R. J., Miller, S. I., and Reed, G. (1980) Alcohol Abuse during

Pregnancy: An Epidemiologic Study. *Alcoholism: Clinical and Experimental Research* **4** (2): 135–45.

Sokol, R. J., Miller, S. I., Debanne, S., Golden, N., Collins, G., Kaplan, J., and Martier, S. (1981) The Cleveland NIAAA Prospective Alcohol-in-Pregnancy Study: The First Year. *Neurobehavioral Toxicology and Teratology* **3**: 203–9.

Spacks, P. M. (1976) *The Female Imagination*. London: Allen & Unwin.

Sparks, S. N. (1984) Speech and Language in Fetal Alcohol Syndrome. *ASHA* **26** February: 2: 27–31.

Spender, D. (1982) *Invisible Women: The Schooling Scandal*. London: Writers and Readers Publishing Co-operative Society.

—— (ed.) (1983) *Feminist Theorists*. London: The Women's Press.

—— (1983) *There's Always Been A Women's Movement This Century*. London: Routledge & Kegan Paul.

Sprent, P. (1979) *Statistics in Action*. Harmondsworth: Penguin Books.

Stacey, M. (ed.) (1976) The Sociology of the NHS. *Sociological Review Monograph* **22**.

Stacey, M. and Price, M. (1981) *Women, Power and Politics*. London: Tavistock.

Staisey, N. L. and Fried, P. A. (1983) Relationships between Moderate Maternal Alcohol Consumption during Pregnancy and Infant Neurological Development. *Journal Studies Alcohol* **44** (2): 262–70.

Stanley, L. and Wise, S. (1983) *Breaking Out: Feminist Consciousness and Feminist Research*. London: Routledge & Kegan Paul.

Steeg, O. N. and Woolf, P. (1979) Cardiovascular Malformations in the Fetal Alcohol Syndrome. *American Heart Journal* **98** (5): 635–37.

Stein, Z. and Kline, J. (1983) Smoking, Alcohol and Reproduction (editorial). *American Journal of Public Health* **73** (10): 1154–156.

Stimmel, B. (ed.) (1982) *The Effects of Maternal Alcohol and Drug Abuse in the Newborn*. Advances in Alcohol and Substance Abuse 1: (3/4). New York: Haworth Press.

Stimpson, C. R. and Person, E. S. (eds) (1980) *Women: Sex and Sexuality*. Chicago, Ill.: The University of Chicago Press.

Stockard, C. R. (1913) The Effect on the Offspring of Intoxicating the Male Parent and the Transmission of the Defects to Subsequent Generations. *American Naturalist* **47**: 641–82.

—— (1924) Alcohol: A Factor in Eliminating Racial Degeneracy. *American Journal Medical Science* **167**: 469–77.

Stockard, C. R. and Papanicolaou, G. (1916) A Further Analysis of the Hereditary Transmission of Degeneracy and Deformities by the Descendants of the Alcoholized Mammals. *American Naturalist* **50** (65–88): 144–77.

Stone, J. L., Smith, H. T., and Murphy, L. B. (eds) (1974) *The Competent Infant*. London: Tavistock.

Strachey, R. (1979) (first published 1928) *The Cause: A Short History of the*

Women's Movement in Great Britain. London: Virago.

Streissguth, A. P. (1976) Maternal Alcoholism and the Outcome of Pregnancy. In M. Greenblatt and M. A. Schuckit (eds) *Alcohol Problems in Women and Children*. New York: Grune & Stratton.

—— (1976) Psychologic Handicaps in Children with Fetal Alcohol Syndrome: Work in Progress on Alcoholism. *New York Academy of Science* **273**: 140–45.

—— (1977) Maternal Drinking and the Outcome of Pregnancy: Implications for Child Mental Health. *American Journal of Orthopsychiatry* **47**: 422–31.

—— (1983) Alcohol and Pregnancy: An Overview and an Update. *Substance Alcohol Action Misuse*: **4** (2–3): 149–73.

Streissguth, A. P., Barr, H. M., Martin, D. C., and Herman, C. S. (1980) Effects of Maternal Alcohol, Nicotine, and Caffeine Use During Pregnancy on Infant Development at Eight Months. *Alcoholism: Clinical and Experimental Research* 4 April 2: 152–63.

Streissguth, A. P., Barr, H. M., and Martin, D. C. (1982) Offspring Effects and Pregnancy Complications Related to Self-Reported Maternal Alcohol Use. *Developmental Pharmacology and Therapeutics* 5: 21–32.

Streissguth, A. P., Martin, D. C., and Buffington, V. E. (1976) Test-Retest Reliability of Three Scales Deriving from a Quantity-Frequency-Variability Assessment of Self-Reported Alcohol Consumption. In F. Seixas (ed.) *Work In Progress in Alcoholism*. New York: Annals of the New York Academy of Sciences **273**: 458–66.

Streissguth, A. P., Martin, D. C., and Buffington, V. E. (1977) Identifying Heavy Drinkers: A Comparison of Eight Alcohol Scores Obtained on the Same Sample. In F. A. Seixas (ed.) *Currents in Alcoholism Vol. II*. New York: Grune & Stratton.

Streissguth, A. P., Martin, D. C., Martin, J. C., and Barr, H. M. (1981) The Seattle Longitudinal Prospective Study on Alcohol and Pregnancy. *Neurobehavioral Toxicology and Teratology* 3: 223–33.

Streissguth, A. P. and Martin, J. C. (1983) Prenatal Effects of Alcohol Abuse in Humans and Laboratory Animals. In B. Kissin and H. Begleiter (eds) *The Pathogenesis of Alcoholism 7*. New York and London: Plenum Press.

Streissguth, A. P., Martin, J. C., and Martin, D. C. (1978) Experimental Design Considerations and Methodological Problems in the Study of the Effects of Social Drinking on the Outcome of Pregnancy. *University of Washington Alcoholism and Drug Abuse Institute Technical Report*: 78–81.

Strickland, D. E. (1984) Content and Effects of Alcohol Advertising. *Journal of Studies on Alcohol* January 45 (1): 87–93.

Strube, G. (1980) *A Woman's Health*. London: Croom Helm.

Sullivan, W. C. (1899) A Note on the Influence of Maternal Inebriety on the Offspring. *Journal of Mental Science* **45**: 489–503.

Sutker, P. A., Libet, J. M., Allain, A. N., and Randeall, C. L. (1983) Alcohol Use, Negative Mood States, and Menstrual Cycle Phases. *Alcoholism* (New York) **7** (3): 327–31.

Swanberg, K. M. and Crumpacker, D. W. (1977) Genetic Differences in Reproductive Fitness and Offspring Viability in Mice Exposed to Alcohol During Gestation. *Behavioral Biology* **20**: 122–27.

Swinscow, T. D. V. (1981) *Statistics at Square One*. London: British Medical Association.

Tanaka, H., Arima, M., and Suzuki, N. (1981) The Fetal Alcohol Syndrome in Japan. *Brain Development* **3**: 305–11.

Taylor, D. (1981) *Alcohol: Reducing the Harm*. London: Office of Health Economics.

Taylor, P. R. (1984) *Smoke Ring: The Politics of Tobacco*. London: The Bodley Head.

Tenbrinck, H. S., and Buchin, S. Y. (1975) Fetal Alcohol Syndrome. *Journal of the American Medical Association* **232**: 1144.

Tennes, K. and Blackard, C. (1980) Maternal Alcohol Consumption, Birth Weight and Minor Physical Anomalies. *American Journal of Obstetrics and Gynecology* **138**: 774–80.

Thompson, W. (1983) (first published 1825) *Appeal of One-half of the Human Race, Women, Against the Pretensions of the Other Half, Men, to Retain Them in Political, and Thence in Civil and Domestic Slavery*. London: Virago.

Thorley, A. (1982) Effects of Alcohol. In M. A. Plant (ed.) *Drinking and Problem Drinking*. London: Junction Books.

Tittmar, H. G. (1982) Statistical Consideration in Analysis of Data in Teratology. Preview of E. L. Abel (ed.) *Fetal Alcohol Syndrome Volume 3 Animal Studies*. Boca Raton, Fla.: CRC Press.

Townsend, P. (1983) *Poverty in the United Kingdom*. Harmondsworth: Penguin Books Ltd.

Townsend, P. and Davidson, N. (1982) *Inequalities in Health: The Black Report*. Harmondsworth: Penguin Books.

Tredrea, D. (1983) (Unpublished) 'What Price the Next Drink?'

Trotter, T. (1813) *An Essay, Medical, Philosophical and Chemical on Drunkenness, and its Effects on the Human Body*. Boston, Mass.: Bradford & Read. (Republished 1981, New York: Arno Press.)

Turner, T. B., Bennett, V. L., and Hernandez, H. (1981) The Beneficial Side of Moderate Alcohol Use. *The Johns Hopkins Medical Journal* **148**: 53–63.

Tze, W. J. and Lee, M. (1975) Adverse Effects of Maternal Alcohol Consumption on Pregnancy Foetal Growth in Rats. *Nature* **257**: 479.

Tze, W. J., Friesen, N. G., and MacLeod, P. K. (1976) Growth Hormone Response in FAS. *Archives of the Diseases of Childhood* **51**: 703–6.

Ulleland, C. N. (1972) The Offspring of Alcoholic Mothers. *Annals New York Academy of Science* **197**: 167–69.

Ulleland, C., Wennberg, R. P., Igo, R. P., and Smith, N. J. (1970) The Offspring of Alcoholic Mothers. *Pediatric Resident* **4**: 474.

United States Department of Commerce (1980) Rising Infant Mortality in the USSR in the 1970s. *International Population Reports.* Series P-95: No. 74.

United States Department of Health, Education and Welfare (1977) *Health Caution in Fetal Alcohol Syndrome.* June.

United States Surgeon General (1981) Advisory on Alcohol and Pregnancy. *Food and Drug Administration Bulletin* **1** (2): 9–10.

Valimaki, M., Harkonen, M., and Ylikahri, R. (1983) Acute Effects of Alcohol on Female Sex Hormones. *Alcoholism* (New York) **7** (3): 289–93.

Van Biervliet, J. P. (1977) The Foetal Alcohol Syndrome. *Acta Paediatrica Belgique* **30** (2): 113–16.

Veghelyi, P. V. and Osztovics, M. (1979) Fetal Alcohol Syndrome in a Child whose Parents had Stopped Drinking. *Lancet* July: 35–6.

Veghelyi, P. V., Osztovics, M., Kardos, G., Leisztner, L., Szaszovszky, E., Igali, S., and Imrei, J. (1978) The Fetal Alcohol Syndrome: Symptoms and Pathogenesis. *Acta Paediatrica Academiae Scientiarum Hungaricae* **19** (3): 171–89.

Vernyt and Kelly, J. (1982) *The Secret Life of the Unborn Child.* London: Sphere Books.

Vogel-Sprott, M. (1983) Response Measures of Social Drinking. Research Implications and Applications. *Journal of Studies on Alcohol* **44** (5): 817–36.

Volicer, B. J., Volicer, L., and D'Angelo, N. (1983) Variation in Length of Time to Development of Alcoholism by Family History of Problem Drinking. *Drug and Alcohol Dependence* **12** (1): 69–83.

Waldrop, M. F. and Halverson, C. F. (1971) Minor Physical Anomalies and Hyperactive Behavior in Young Children. In J. Hellmuth (ed.) *The Exceptional Infant vol. II.* New York: Bruner Mogel.

Walsh, A. C. (1977) Dangers of Minimal Drinking (Letter). *American Journal of Psychiatry* **134** (9): 1049–50.

Waltman, R. and Iniquez, E. S. (1972) Placental Transfer of Ethanol and its Elimination at Term. *Obstetrics and Gynecology* **40** (2): 180–85.

Wandor, M. (ed.) (1978) *The Body Politic.* London: Stage I.

Warner, R. H. and Rosett, H. L. (1975). The Effects of Drinking on Offspring. *Journal of Studies on Alcohol* **36** (11): 1395–420.

Warren, K. (ed.) (1977) A Critical Review of the Fetal Alcohol Syndrome. Presented at the NIAAA Press Conference, Washington DC, 1 June.

Warren, K. R. and Rosett, H. L. (1978) FAS: New Perspectives. *Alochol Health and Research World* **24**: 2–12.

Weideger, P. (1977) *Female Cycles.* London: The Women's Press.

Weiner, L., Rosett, H. L., Edelin, K. C., Alpert, J. J., and Zuckermann, B. (1983) Alcohol Consumption by Pregnant Women. *Obstetrics and Gynaecology* **61**: 6–12.

Whitlock, F. A. (1975) Alcoholism: A Genetic Disorder? *Australia and New Zealand Journal of Psychiatry* 9 (1): 3–7.
Williams, C. D. and Jelliffe, D. B. (1978) *Mother and Child Health: Delivering the Services.* Oxford: Oxford University Press.
Williams, D. L., Maclean, A. W., and Cairns, J. (1983) Dose-Response Effects of Ethanol on the Sleep of Young Women. *Journal Studies Alcohol* 44 (3): 515–23.
Williams, G. P. and Brake, G. T. (1980) *Drink in Great Britain 1900 to 1979.* London: B. Edsall.
Wilson, A. (1982) *The Wise Virgin: The Missing Link between Men and Women.* Wellingborough, Northamptonshire: Turnstone Press.
Wilson, K. H., Landesman, R., Fuchs, A. R., and Fuchs, F. (1969) The Effect of Ethyl Alcohol on Isolated Human Myometruim. *American Journal of Obstetrics and Gynecology* 104: 436–39.
Wilson, M. (1981) Personal communication.
Wilson, P. (1980a) *Drinking in England and Wales.* London: HMSO.
—— (1980b) Drinking Habits in the United Kingdom. *Population Trends.* Winter: 14–18. London: HMSO.
Woollam, D. H. M. (1978) F.A.S. as an Example of Mammilian Teratology. *All Faith's World Alcohol Project Journal* 1.
—— (1981) Alcohol and the Safety of the Unborn Child. *Royal Society of Health Journal* 6: 241–44.
Worsley, P. (ed.) (1977) *Introducing Sociology: Second Edition.* Harmondsworth: Penguin Books.
—— (ed.) (1980) *Modern Sociology: Second Edition.* Harmondsworth: Penguin Books.
Wright, E. (1978) *The New Childhood.* London: W. H. Allen.
Wright, E. (1964) *The New Childbirth.* London: Universal Tandem.
Wright, H. (1981) *Swallow it Whole: The New Statesman's Survival Guide to the Food Industry.* London: New Statesman.
Wright, J. H. (1981) Fetal Alcohol Syndrome: The Social Work Connection. *Health and Social Work* February 6 (1): 5–10.
Wright, J. T., Barrison, I. G., Lewis, I. G., Macrae, K. D., Waterson, E. J., Toplis, P. J., Gordon, M. G., and Morris, N. F. (1983) Alcohol Consumption, Pregnancy and Low Birth Weight. *Lancet* March: 663–65.
Wright Mills, C. (1980) *The Sociological Imagination.* Harmondsworth: Pelican Books.
Zur Linden, W. (1980) *A Child is Born: Pregnancy, Birth, Early Childhood.* London: Rudolf Steiner Press.

Name index

Subject index

166